AUTHOR'S NOTE

All of the events described in this book are real. They were assembled in tape-recorded interviews with the people named and from my memories of events I have witnessed or heard described on a first-person basis.

Some of the people interviewed asked that their identities be obscured. In those cases I have either simply changed names or, when the facts of someone's experience would pinpoint his or her identity, I have converted facts to similar facts in order to protect the privacy of the people involved.

In the case of my memories, I have tried to be as accurate as time and the colorings of intervening events will allow.

MISCARRIAGE

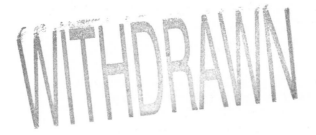

Simon & Brown

For information on bulk orders, please contact
info@simonandbrown.com *or go to*
www.simonandbrown.com

Miscarriage

ISBN 978-0-9814843-2-7

Library of Congress Control Number: 2008932356
Library of Congress subject headings:
Miscarriage – Psychological Aspects
Miscarriage – Psychological Aspects – Case Studies
Bereavement– Psychological Aspects
Bereavement– Psychological Aspects – Case Studies

1.0

By the Grace of God
this book is dedicated to
Tucker Jennings Williamson
May she never need it
And may she come to be
proud of it.
With Love, from
her father

ACKNOWLEDGEMENTS

First let me thank the people who opened their lives and their pain to me. Not only did they make this book plausible; they made it possible.

Carol Anderson had read some of the material that became the last two chapters and she sent me to Beth Walker. I thank them both.

Ann Dewey made one of the interviews possible and encouraged me all along the way. And Elizabeth Fielding, Barli Wakefield, Gin Taylor McClure, and especially April Keech were of unflagging support.

Hal, Robert, Susan, Rocco, Maria, and a host of other friends read and reread chapters and commented, bolstered, and comforted. Debby Parker was my most loyal and faithful reader, as she has been a loyal and faithful friend.

My editor, Barbara Ravage, has shown patience and wisdom and unfailing taste and knowledge.

CONTENTS

Introduction

"**B**arbara has gone into labor."

If the message had come some months later it would have created great joy and celebration. But Barbara was only in the fifth month of her pregnancy. She had been having trouble from the beginning. Now it was clear. She was losing the baby.

I was at my table editing a piece on a child actor in a Broadway show. The sitter had our daughter in the park. I reached for the phone again.

"Mrs. Williamson is in a meeting." We have an agreement: She does not call during nap time; I do not interrupt meetings.

"Would you tell her that this is her husband and that I would like to speak with her now, please." My tone was sharper than I had planned, but it was effective. In a moment Sam, my wife, was on the line.

"What's the matter?" She knew that I would not breech the agreement without good cause.

"Barbara has gone into labor. They called from church. She's at the hospital. I thought you would want to know."

"You were right to call." There was a long pause. We were both afraid to say too much. Our days were busy, and this was no time to weaken.

"I wish we could be together to pray."

"So do I."

It was not until later, after the phone calls and the half-hearted attempt to pray alone and the refilled coffee mug and the sitting quietly trying to pull myself together, that it struck. A wave of ugly bitter emptiness welled up in me, and I found myself sobbing with a violent grief I had not known for many months—not since the last time some accident of information had opened that closed door of my memory and brought me face to face with our first child, the one who died before it was born.

In the months since Barbara's miscarriage, and to a certain extent in the years since our own, I have forced myself to think a lot about the subject. I have done so because my own experience and the experiences of many around me have led me to believe that to avoid putting the issue into perspective is to keep the wound that is miscarriage open and unhealed. If that wound can begin to heal, if the running sore of pain can be staunched and sealed—understood and accepted—then it may cause scars, but it will cease to infect the rest of life.

Those people who have not known this kind of death may think I am being melodramatic to speak of wounds and infection and death. After all, they reason, we're not talking about a person who died. We're talking about a . . . well, not a person. It was a medical event, wasn't it? It was something that didn't happen, not something that did. It was a physical mistake, an accident, a nonevent. Such thinking is wrong and insensitive. It is also understandable.

I was sitting with a wise friend, a doctor, when it struck me. "I'm beginning to think," I said, "that no one who has not been there can truly understand what miscarriage is." He smiled. He was aware of my work on this book. He nodded slowly and said, "You may be right. It's like cancer, or amputation, or any of those horrors. You can be sympathetic. But you cannot truly understand it until it has happened to you." I did not want to believe that. I did not want to believe that it was a case of Us versus Them. And yet in almost every situation I had studied there had been an element of loneliness and estrangement, a sense that no one could see or recognize the depth of the pain. Friends and family could be patient and kind. Doctors and counselors could be open and resourceful. But there were still gaps, still places in the pain that remained isolated and raw. In many cases the only solace that came close to those places was from the people who had their own miscarriage wounds and scars.

On the other hand, there was ample evidence of impatience, insensitivity, and dismissal, even from those people who one would think would know better. Parents, doctors, counselors were sometimes too quick to move past the trauma without giving the victims, or indeed themselves, enough space to absorb and understand what had happened. Those attitudes further complicated the already tangled web of feelings and emotions that seemed to trap the people who had been hurt. And they added subtly to the inevitable sense of isolation felt by any victim of any trauma.

Perhaps, I began to think, the best way to help both the people who suffer and the people who try to help them is simply to lay out the experiences, the facts, and the observations I had come to or gathered. That, then, is what I have done.

I am not an expert. I believe that there are no experts where miscarriage is concerned. I am simply a person who has suffered and watched suffering. My observations are not always objective, for they have been filtered through those unique experiences each of us uses to inform our vision and sort out our perceptions. I have tried to be logical, and it is with logic that we should begin this or any such journey.

Logic, whether conscientiously applied or instinctively perceived, tells us that there has been life here and now it is gone. That is called death.

There is some power, some force, some electrochemical activity that invests flesh with individuality and definition.

When it is present, whether the entity is self-determining or, like a fetus, mother-dependent, it is alive. When that power is gone the flesh has no more personhood or individuality than a filet of sole packed on ice. I ask for no factual explanation of it. I simply know that the difference between life and death has to do with the presence or absence of that power.

Why then, I wonder, should we continue to try to distinguish between the kind of grief we feel at the death of a person who lasted long enough to acquire a name and the kind that at least one person I talked to in the course of writing this book called "unsuitable grief." The sense of that phrase was that the dead fetus was not a person, not alive, not an individual, so the mother and father were simply being self-indulgent to let their grief last for longer than a few weeks. I have news for those who hold that view: Death is death. Whether it comes at the end of a long and full span of living or before that span has even begun, the flesh that housed a person is now empty and we must grieve for that emptiness.

Most of us try to keep death at a distance. When someone very close to us dies we are profoundly affected. When we hear of the death of a distant friend we are less moved. And when we read of the death of a public figure or mass death in a faraway war or natural cataclysm we say, "Isn't that awful," and turn the page. The degree to which we are involved with a death is a direct function of the degree to which we were involved with the life of the deceased. And we like it that way. We can manage death that way. If we do not know the person we can limit our vulnerability to the grief that must surely follow the event. Yet in miscarriage we have both the most intimate involvement and the greatest distancing. We are physically involved in the most direct and tactile way. But we never knew a name, never saw a smile, never heard a laugh. Our knowledge of this being is a reversal of the norm. We know our physical proximity best by the effects on the mother, not by an awareness of the child. And we have invested a wealth of emotion in a person we have never met, have not shared with, and will have neither mementos nor memories of.

The problem with miscarriage is that it defies our usual ways of ordering life. There are certain distinctions that miscarriage bypasses. We cannot say that we knew this baby in the same way we can say that we knew a born person. And yet we knew this baby well. We cannot say this baby died, because by our accepted definitions death involves a distinguishable person and an agreed-upon set of end signs and ceremonies. And yet this baby died. In a society that sanctions abortion it is socially risky to say that this baby was ever alive. And yet we know that there was life here and now it is gone.

What then can we say about miscarriage?

We can say that it is frequent. Statistically, miscarriage seems to be on the increase. One estimate places the number at about 20 percent of all pregnancies, or about three hundred thousand each year in the United States. There is also some evidence that a great many missed or late menstrual periods were actually conceptions that miscarried. Beyond the numbers, however, is the fact that it is almost impossible to mention miscarriage in a group of people without one or more acknowledging their own losses.

I had the delightful experience several years before her death of appearing in a play with Vivian Vance. She had had, only a year or so before, a radical mastectomy for breast cancer. I was helping her with her costumes and so we ended up discussing her operation at some length. She was frank about the procedure itself and the limitations it placed on the way she dressed and the strength of her arm. But during our talks she brought up several times the fact that as soon as word got out she was overwhelmed by women she knew who had had the same operation. "They just came out of the woodwork," said Viv. "People I had known for years and had worked with closely were suddenly telling me that they had been through the same thing, and I never knew about it."

Miscarriage is like that. It does not show. It is not something you want to talk about at a party. There is no evidence of it in your home. It remains unspoken, unknown, and so, unacknowledged, until some chance remark or urgent need calls it forth. Ironically, one of the best tools of recovery is the talking, the revealing, the very sharing that rarely takes place simply because the need is not seen or appreciated.

Another thing that can be said about miscarriage is that no one knows how to deal with it well. Because of the limbo status to which circumstance consigns it, miscarriage is in some ways more enduring than an ordinary death. There is no ending to it because it never really began—according to our accepted rules of beginning. Most of the time we do not even see the fetus, so our mourning seems to be for a nothing, a fiction, an invisible phantom. The most many of us get to look at is an image on a sonograph screen, and all too often that image is too still and too small to allow us to rejoice at the marvelous technology that lets us see inside the womb. Too often the technicians are too technical. Too often the report is too objective.

Then there are the guilt games we play with ourselves. What if I had done this differently? What if I had not done that? What if I had called, had asked, had taken, had not eaten, what if, what if, what if? To all that is now added a guilty conflict over what constitutes life: viability or simply life itself?

Often other people grow impatient with our grief. They have not known our dead. They have often not recognized the dead as a person. They cannot understand why this essentially medical phenomenon should cause such a trauma. They are sympathetic to us as friends, but usually they have trouble identifying with our dead child as a person. That puts a strain on our willingness to accept their comforting.

When I was in high school my drama teacher was as much friend as mentor. When her mother died several of us took turns spending time with Ms. K., hoping to ease the loneliness and loss. With the best intentions, we were trying to distract her. But we found that what she really needed was to pay attention to her grief, to talk about her mother. She told us stories about her childhood and described her mother's likes and tastes. She wanted to keep her mother clear in her memory while the shock and pain began to heal. When ordinary death has touched me since, I have experienced the wisdom of her example. When I have been grieved I have needed more than anything else friends who would simply be there to listen. Unfortunately, in the case of miscarriage there are no memories to share, and few people, no matter how close or well intentioned, have the patience to simply be still and available. Most want to do something. There is nothing to be done. Most want to say something. There is nothing to be said.

Miscarriage is a different class of death. It has all the trauma and ugliness of ordinary death with none of death's sense of completion or fulfillment. It bypasses the memories and the shared experiences. It leaves out the layers of involvement, the growth of relationship, the bonds of living and loving. Miscarriage is just all the bad parts.

But miscarriage does get better. It never truly goes away, but it does get better. That seems to be one of the only good things miscarriage shares with ordinary death. Time and patience, compassion and perspective will eventually incorporate miscarriage into the body of our experience and allow us to go on living. That does not happen quickly and it does not happen easily. But it can happen.

Current understanding describes grief as more a process than a single emotion, a series of stages through which the victim passes on the way to healthy resolution. In simplified form, first there is shock. We want to deny, to control, to freeze the action. Events and emotions appear to be flying

9

in all directions and we cannot seem to manage our own minds anymore. Then comes pain. We blame ourselves, we flatten out our highs in the hope of drawing up our lows, we get angry and solemn in the same moment. We feel as if we are afloat in a dismal gray sea of cold soft misery. Finally we begin to heal, to accept, to put into perspective. We begin to displace death with living.

We come into contact with many people during these stages. Our reaction to them (and their reaction to us) is based on both our current stage of healing and our expectations of what they can mean to our healing process. Yet, it is likely that we will make as many mistakes in our expectations of what these people can provide as they will make mistakes in how they manifest their care.

When Richard and Barbara, our friends, miscarried in the fifth month of their first pregnancy, my wife and I found that we could help. Sam spent some time just sitting with Barbara, letting her know that she was not alone. Sam knew exactly the kinds of thoughts and feelings Barbara was experiencing. I was able to comfort Richard some for the same reasons. I had been there. They were also helped by others who had not been there but had taken the time and care to recognize the depth of the pain and the complexity of the road to healing.

For Sam and me it had been the successful birth of our daughter that finally left us little room for grief. For others it may be work, or recognizing love, or simply coming to terms with the reality of what has happened that finally closes the door on the trauma.

It was out of sharing our story, our pain, and our healing with Barbara and Richard, and letting them share theirs with us, that this book was born. I hope that by sharing our two stories and the others that are recorded here—stories and thoughts and observations—I can help other victims of miscarriage, as well as those who attend them as they make their way through this different class of death.

1

Barbara and Richard

N

o one had warned her. She was totally unprepared for this. She awoke at four in the morning on Friday in the hospital and the whole front of her gown was wet. Her breasts were very sore and felt like footballs. And no one had warned her. Her body did not know that the baby was dead, had been dead since Tuesday. So her body had gone ahead and produced the milk that was supposed to nourish the baby. It was adding insult to injury. Finally Barbara cried. Finally, after being brave and hopeful and even a little proud of herself for surviving the delivery, there alone in the middle of the night the full weight of what had happened set in and she cried with the heartbreak that only a mother who has lost her child can know.

It was an "iffy" pregnancy from the beginning: four years of trying crowned by a conception that started with bleeding and cramps. She quit her job, and the doctor put her to bed for two of the first four months. Now, in the fifth month, she had been given a clean bill of health. A well-meaning friend had commented only last week, "You couldn't get that kid out now with dynamite."

Sunday night she started spotting. On the doctor's orders she stayed in bed all day Monday. Then, before dawn on Tuesday, Barbara was awakened by cramps. Richard, her husband, was groggy but aware that she could not get back to sleep, and at 6:00 A.M. he heard her nausea turn to violent dry vomiting. After that Barbara noticed that the cramping was following a pattern almost like the descriptions she had read of . . . But this could not be labor. She was only in the fifth month—the twenty-first week.

By nine the pains were closer together. She and Richard went to the doctor's office. The doctor took one look and sent them to the hospital. She told them to go directly to the floor, but when they got there the nurse stopped them. Hadn't they been admitted? Then she took a second look at Barbara. Quietly she told Richard to go downstairs and do the paperwork; she would put Barbara to bed right away.

The pain was getting worse, and more regular. Richard was back now. Barbara's mother had come. The resident was in and out, as was the nurse. Richard had called the church and a prayer tree had been started. All over the city people were praying for them. But Barbara knew what was happening.

By noon Barbara told the resident that she was not getting any relief at all between contractions. He said that that was good, that she would probably deliver within the next ten to fifteen minutes. He left her room to prepare for the procedure. No sooner had the door closed than Barbara felt a new kind of movement and the pain stopped. She told her mother, who looked under the covers and confirmed the baby's arrival. Richard dashed into the hall and dragged the doctor back. For a moment all was quiet. The fetal heartbeat had stopped some time before, but Barbara finally got up the courage to ask how it looked.

"Is there anything apparently wrong with it?"

"No," said the doctor, "It looks just fine."

"Is it a boy or a girl?" asked Barbara.

Richard answered. "It's a little boy." His voice was steady but slightly hushed.

Finally Barbara ventured into the area that would turn mere sensation into fact. "May I see him?"

With the care one would use in lifting fine crystal, the

doctor moved the cord so that the baby could be brought into view. He was tiny but perfectly formed, with long delicate hands and transparent skin, and to Barbara's eyes he was beautiful. "Okay," thought Barbara with the same humor that had sustained her through the times of doubt. "We have a good recipe. Now we just need to keep it in the oven a little longer."

Barbara had lost a lot of blood. The D and C that was necessary to remove the placenta took more. She was weak, but her spirits were good. They had gotten halfway through. They would try again and make it all the way. And with all the pain and fear and doubt, she had survived. That made her feel better. Wednesday and Thursday she had been objective and brave. Then Friday morning she woke up with the lactation, and the crying started. The full impact of what had happened became a fixed reality. And as they were leaving the hospital the elevator door opened on the maternity floor. There was a couple taking their new baby home. It was like a slap in the face. Richard and Barbara both felt it. It was the start of a journey of healing that would take many months and, as they have realized, may never really be completed.

On a cold clear Sunday afternoon in December, some six months after the event, I sat with Richard and Barbara in their cozy apartment. Richard was serving warm cider in delicate china and around the fireplace the records and tapes and books and artwork that would have been Gabe's environment spoke of a well-read, sensitive, musical, devout, appreciative family. Gabe was their nickname for their not-born son.

"I was removed from it to a degree," said Richard, recalling the moment the doctor called him over to see that the baby was already descending. "I was very clinical. 'Yes, I can see what you mean. . . . Yes, okay, we'll go to the hospital now.' It was happening, but it was happening to

15

Barbara. She was in pain. She was the one it was happening to. It wasn't until she had had the baby and I saw it that I felt involved at all. This was my child too. Up until then it was 'my wife is hurting.'"

Ironically, it was Richard who experienced the first tears. Tall and trim, with thinning, prematurely silver hair, Richard is an executive at a large university. After they got to the hospital he called his office to say that he would not be in. ". . . to tell the office manager that Barbara was in the hospital, and I said, 'She's losing the baby.' Having to say that . . ." His voice slows and quiets and thickens a bit even today. "Having to really say that . . . that hurt."

Barbara, small with dark, dark hair and pale, pale skin, tells of their arrival at home. Before they even put her to bed she gathered up a diary of letters she had been writing to the baby and carried them to the fireplace. As the pages burned Barbara found herself crying. Looking into the mirror she saw that Richard was standing behind her crying too. Finally removed from the public pressure of the hospital they were able to share their loss fully and in private for the very first time.

"I don't think I ever had a clue how critical the loss would be," says Barbara. "No matter how career-oriented you may be, everything in your life gets shifted and the role of 'mama' becomes central to everything in your being. I'm a good writer. I write a lot. People seek me out to write for them. But after the miscarriage I felt totally worthless. I was a failure at what I was supposed to do."

Richard adds, "And there was nothing I could do. My supportive-husband thing didn't work, and everything I said sounded hollow."

Barbara is frank to admit thoughts of suicide. Her life seemed to have no value. Her mother, raised in another generation, did not understand. "Oh, don't be silly!" was not what Barbara needed to hear. It was a wise friend who

16

had been through the same thing who explained to Barbara that the hormonal storms of postpartum adjustment would go on for a couple of months and that the emotional and psychological adjustment would take even longer. Barbara began to recognize the difference between the emotional and the chemical, and on days when "a short ledge on the thirty-fifth floor" looked good she was able to tell herself not "Oh, that's silly," but "Oh, that's my hormones."

Barbara was in bed at home for three weeks before she was allowed a short walk around the neighborhood. Although they lived in a lovely area thick with stately townhouses and trees and elegant shops, Barbara saw three things only on her outing: a pregnant woman, one baby in a stroller, and another in a summer Snugli. She arrived home as if chased and breathed a sigh of relief that she had not embarrassed herself on the street by breaking down in tears.

Talking about the things that trigger the grief, Barbara can be a bit more objective today. "Those triggers, they come from nowhere," she says.

"And they're not necessarily what you'd expect," adds Richard. "Barbara came across the photograph of the sonogram of the baby the other day, and it was fine."

"Yeah," she confirms, "it was fine. I want to keep that. But I walked into the kitchen one day and there was this little clay bowl I've had since my childhood and . . ." Her voice breaks off. After a moment she continues talking with her eyes going red and her smile fixed as a weapon to fight off the tears. "And then there are those times when you're not thinking about it at all and it suddenly just wells up. You think 'I'm not in control' and you start to wonder if you'll ever be in control again."

For the most part Richard and Barbara praise the counsel they got from friends and family. They were told to be patient with themselves. They were told to take one day at a time. They were told to recognize that they had been through a major trauma, and to give themselves time and space to grieve, fully and with no pretense of bravery or false self-control.

The number of people who have come forward to say that they, too, have had the awful experience has astonished them. Knowing that helps since most of those people now have healthy children. "It's almost like a prerequisite. Or that's the way it seems sometimes," says Barbara.

The most helpful friends kept calling and coming by. They realized that the healing would take a long time. And they only got one classic "It was God's will." Richard and Barbara, deeply devout, do not believe that God works that way. But Barbara cringes at the line she used to use to comfort friends: "You'll have another one." Today she knows that her own answer to such a glib remark would be: "I don't want another one. I want that one."

Richard serves another round of mulled cider while Barbara talks about the fear and guilt that set in a few weeks after she got home from the hospital. She was plagued with thoughts that perhaps this had been their only chance, or that something inside her had been damaged by the medical procedures. And she could not shake the thought that something she had done might have contributed to the miscarriage. Item by item she reviewed for her doctor every step she took, everything she ate and drank. Finally the doctor realized what was going on and looked her squarely in the eye. "Barbara," she said, "You are not responsible for this miscarriage," and proceeded to look for the true cause of the loss.

The doctor suspected that the problem may have been what is called an incompetent cervix. If that were the case then there was a simple and effective treatment involving a stitch to seal the opening until the baby was fully ready. The possibility that something could be done helped lift Barbara out of her depression. At the same time her former boss called to say that she wanted Barbara back on any basis.

Both self-worth and hope began to return. The testing would have to wait until Barbara's period resumed and had been followed through two cycles. This gave Barbara some time to rebuild confidence and objectivity. But when the test had been run the results were inconclusive and Barbara was plunged back into depression for a time. She seemed to be going right back to the same situation she had been in before with nothing having been done to keep it all from happening again.

Yet, her inventory of assets began to emerge. She had a loving husband, a comfortable home, and friends who had proven themselves in time of crisis. Her faith in God had been temporarily shaken but that, too, had proven to be an expected part of the healing process. And He had been patient with her. "The thing that was so important was the love. Just love. The best help was the people who didn't try to say it would be better. It wouldn't be better. They were honest. So they just listened to us. And loved us."

The afternoon was waning and the cider had cooled. I started to turn off my tape recorder when Barbara said, "You know, it's funny. Now that we're trying again, every time we've made love I've had a sense that Gabe was there, cheering us on." It is a lovely thought.

As I waited for a taxi in the cold December wind I knew that Barbara and Richard would be all right. They understand their scars. They are surrounded by faith and love and hope. And, in a way, they still have Gabe. They know that he was once alive. They know that he was their child. And it has become very clear to them that they loved him—not as an idea but as a person.

2

Grandmothers and Sex

S he did not really want to be interviewed. She insisted I not use her name or anything about her that could identify her beyond the fact that her daughter had had a miscarriage. I talked to them both separately and pieced together the story from the little things they said and did not say.

Alice (I'll call her Alice) is sixty-two years old. She was born in the 1920s and came into adulthood during World War II. The Great Depression formed many of her social and personal ideas. She had one older sister, who married and had two children during the late thirties. In 1944 her sister's husband was killed during a training accident at an army base in Kansas. Alice watched her sister struggle to keep her two small children fed and housed until she remarried in the early 1950s. The man she married was kind and stable and provided for his new family with patient and undemanding calm.

Alice married Bob in 1948. She had known him before the war and had gone through the conflict hoping that he would return from his work as an illustrator for army publications stationed in Washington. After the war he got a job with an advertising agency and asked Alice to marry him. Joyce, their daughter, was born in 1952. Joyce was a cherished child and always felt loved and understood by her parents, although as she reached adulthood she and her mother seemed to grow a bit distant from each other.

When Joyce announced that she was going to marry Randall in 1979 both her mother and father were delighted. Randall was in business for himself and quite successful. Bob was impressed by Randall's sense of humor and his love of music and art, and the two men enjoyed discussing exhibits and concerts. Alice wanted Joyce to be happy and well provided for, and Randall seemed to be the answer on both counts.

Two years after the wedding Joyce told her mother that she and Randall had decided to get pregnant. Alice received the news with a noticeable lack of enthusiasm. She first told Joyce to make sure she was not rushing into motherhood before she had fully enjoyed her career and her husband. When Joyce and Randall did not conceive right away Alice comforted her daughter with the fact that at least she would not have to give up her good job as a fashion buyer so soon. Alice concentrated on the practical aspects of the situation. When Joyce grew frustrated by her failure to conceive her mother would grow quiet and a bit impatient.

When Joyce finally did conceive in 1983 her mother smiled a lot but said little. Joyce wanted to tell friends and relatives, but Alice advised waiting until further along. It was just "not a good idea" to announce these things too early. You never knew what might happen. Joyce was puzzled by what she perceived as a lack of joy on her mother's part.

Alice had never been demonstrative. She was kind and gentle, but she was not the more affectionate of Joyce's parents. That title went to Bob, who reinforced Joyce constantly with physical and emotional warmth. When Joyce miscarried in the third month of her pregnancy it was Bob who sat in the room holding her hand and weeping. Alice was there, too. But Alice was obviously uncomfortable and almost immediately began a series of "You've got to get over this" lectures.

It was a week or so after the miscarriage that Alice started again with one of her motherly talks. They were alone for the Saturday afternoon. Bob and Randall were off at an art exhibit. Joyce had been feeling dark and lonely all day. When Alice started Joyce felt a sudden urge to hit her mother. Instead, she looked her in the eye and asked, "Why?" Alice was startled by her daughter's frank confrontation. For a moment she said nothing. Then, for the first time in years, Joyce saw her mother burst into tears. Deep sobs of anguish heaved up and shook her mother's body, and Joyce stood frozen for a moment before rushing to her side and helping her into a chair. As the story unfolded Joyce felt her anger give way to confusion and then to understanding.

In 1950, two years before Joyce was born, Alice had a miscarriage. She and Bob had not been very careful about using the condoms that Bob kept in his dresser drawer. When Alice missed her first period she was delighted and hopeful and said nothing. She wanted to be sure. When she missed her second she made an appointment with her doctor. Bob did not even know that she suspected. He had been busy with a job change and with some traveling, and they were not in the habit of discussing "female complaints." Two days before the doctor's appointment Alice awoke feeling very sluggish. Pressure in her abdomen sent her to the bathroom, where she discovered she was bleeding. Not knowing what to do she did nothing. By midday she was bleeding heavily, and she continued to cramp and gush for the rest of the afternoon and evening. Bob was in Washington working on a project, and Alice stayed alone with a hot water bottle and a towel. By the following day the bleeding was down to the regular spotting she was familiar with. She was fairly sure she knew what had happened and when she went to the doctor the following day he confirmed her suspicion. She ventured only one question, to which the doctor's answer was, "The baby was so small that it probably passed in a clot and you never even knew it." The "spontaneous abortion" was clean and there was no need for a D and C. For more than thirty years only Alice and her doctor knew of the event.

The simple reading of the story holds that Alice had never come to terms with her own miscarriage. Her hesitation over Joyce's marriage and attempts to get pregnant, her paining lack of sympathy for Joyce's trauma can easily be traced to her own ambivalence and unshared grief. Yet there are other layers to this story that need to be explored.

Miscarriage involves several kinds of failure. There is the obvious physiological failure of the baby to grow and develop properly or of the mother's body to sustain the pregnancy. But the sense of failure runs deeper than this.

At one depth there is a failure of expectation. Even at those times when we have avoided pregnancy we have not been able to escape periodic musings over what we might be like as parents, what our own parents would think of our offspring, what it would be like to hold a child of our own in our arms. We have felt the tug of social acceptance both when friends or relatives have said, "When are you two going to start your family?" and when we have seen children being born around us. Then we were pregnant, and the musings and the tugging and the desire to be part of this particular mainstream were suddenly a reality. We could see the physical changes, we could count the actual days and weeks and months, we could anticipate a real baby. Then the baby was dead, the pregnancy was over, and all that investment was lost. The expectations had been wasted along with the baby. It is like paying into a savings account and suddenly finding that the bank has gone out of business.

There is yet another level of failure that is not usually addressed. In addition to being a mechanical failure and a failure of social expectation, miscarriage is, in a very real way, a sexual failure.

Logic tells us that a psychological sequence exists by which we can work backward from *baby* to *conception* to *sex act* to *sexual prowess* to *self-image*. Beginning at the end—*baby*—we can trace one major theme of our concept of parenting backward so that we end at the beginning—*self-image*. In a subtle and important way our children are an extension of our self-image, and one of the principal cords that binds the two is the sex act, not just as a mechanical means of reproduction but as a primary psychological component of the process. A failure of this extension, a failure to parent for whatever reason, becomes a failure of our sexual prowess and a threat to our sexual self-image.

Modern thinking, shaped by advertising, films, television, and much of the popular literature on sex, encourages us to move in only one direction, and only part way at that. We must improve our self-image so that we can improve our sexual prowess so that we can improve our sex act—and we're supposed to stop right there, exhausted and sensually fulfilled. Through the miracles of modern chemistry and latex technology we are able to invoke the doctrine of "sequence interruptus."

I would be the last to denigrate the joy and wonder of pure sensuality or to deny the wisdom of family planning in a world whose economic demands make large families impractical. All I am saying is that chemistry and technology have not altered the basic sequence. No matter how good the health club makes you look or how thin the diet cola keeps your thighs or how sexy your butt looks in your designer jeans, having babies is still a basic psychological component of sexuality and the denial or avoidance of that fact leads to frustration, confusion, and emotional dis-ease.

We rightly feel that we are supposed to be sexual. There is a built-in urge for sex that longs to be satisfied. Celibacy requires inordinate and convoluted sublimation because the body all but demands that we purge our sexual energy periodically. Nature has given us an instinctive desire to couple. It has done this by making sex the most extreme physical pleasure available. And I believe Nature has done this because it knows that we are easily distracted. Without the pleasure component of sex we might well become so involved in making bombs and money that the race would die out altogether.

Because of the pleasure principle we have continued to copulate since the proverbial caveman dragged the proverbial cave woman back to the cave by the hair. But the reason for the pleasure is to insure the copulation and the reason for insuring the copulation is the propagation of the species. It is modern science, the avowed enemy of the secret ways of Nature, that has, through chemistry and technology, made it possible to separate sexual pleasure from sexual purpose. I realize that these thoughts fly in the face of most "up-to-date" thinking. But logic insists that whether you believe in a creative God or in existential randomness, Nature has insured its own survival by making sex, which begins with personal passion and does not really end until that passion has been answered with a 2:00 A.M. feeding, great fun.

Now, why am I giving so much space to this argument? There are two reasons. First, to establish the fact that any social convention, whether it be post-Victorian prudery, which celebrates the reproductive portion of the sequence while denying the pleasure portion, or irresponsible singles-bar hedonism, which reverses that celebration—*any social convention that impedes the natural flow from the pleasure of the bed to the pleasure of the nursery—sets itself against the entire force of Nature.* Second, to establish the fact that an unexpected interruption in that flow—and by that I mean a miscarriage—is not only a personal affront to the sexual prowess and self-image of the individuals involved. It is a failure felt instinctively on a grand scale, pitting the weakness of the puny man and woman against the design and power of the workings of the universe. And if you do not believe this ask someone staring down at a bloody mass of tissue that was once a living fetus how much he or she feels like the master of his or her own fate. When victims of miscarriage speak of feeling like failures that is *exactly* what they mean.

Like most little boys I was taught that I was not supposed to look too closely at my mother naked. But what child has not had the experience of opening a closed door, saying, "Mama, I want a . . . Oh! Excuse me." My sister was born when I was ten. Mother got very fat and someone explained that was where the baby was and that it would come out down where she peed. That made no sense to me at all. The day my sister was born Mother lost her lump so I figured they must have been right about the baby having been in her belly, but I still did not want to think about the coming-out-where-she-peed part.

I grew up in a family that taught that nice people never discussed religion or politics. Sex was so far from *nice* that we did not even discuss the fact that we did not discuss it. When I was twelve my father took half an hour to confirm what I had already learned from the neighborhood boys, with a heavy emphasis on understanding a lot more after I was married. Fortunately, something called the sexual revolution was just beginning. I went to a college that prohibited horizontal socializing, but around the country there were near-naked couples carrying "Make Love Not War" posters through the streets. The Pill was supposed to make all things possible. The many generations of randy teens on whom pregnancy had had a scarecrow effect were now seen as quaint, repressed and foolish.

During those dear, and ironically innocent, days most of us were hungry for the information propriety had denied us at home. We passed around our information, and misinformation, along with our dog-eared copies of the *Kama Sutra* and *The Joy of Sex*. Everyone, it seemed, was obsessed with *doing it* better. Little time or energy went into what to do with the problems of sex. Abortion was not yet a topic of table conversation. It was still essentially a back-street affair, and I was never sure whether the drunken abortionist used his kitchen knife from the inside or the outside because in the stories I heard the girl always died in the end anyway.

Infertility was another issue that was glossed over at the time. A friend who had suffered a severe case of mumps in his youth was not sure until his girlfriend got pregnant whether or not he was capable of fathering a child. At their wedding he told me (with an odd combination of pride in his accomplishment and regret that he would have to be more careful in the future) that if the mumps had been more severe it would have made his life simpler.

Miscarriage was hardly ever mentioned. We all knew that it sometimes happened, but the specifics did not seem to matter back then. When Scarlett O'Hara fell down the staircase it somehow knocked the baby out of her. That was about the extent of our awareness of miscarriage.

Being enthralled with open sexuality and, because of that, feeling superior to our parents' generation, we put an even wider gap between those of us who reached maturity in the sixties and seventies and those who had come to adulthood some twenty or thirty years earlier. We thought, with some justification, that We understood *doing it* and They did not. We distanced ourselves from our parents over sex as we did over Viet Nam and race and all the other issues of the politically charged public arena of the time. What we failed to recognize then, and what we continue to pay dearly for in feelings of estrangement and isolation, is the power of the sequence that binds our psychology to our biology. The very sexuality we were claiming as our own independent turf was holding us fast to the generation we were claiming independence from.

There are two reasons why all of this is important to our understanding of miscarriage. One is simply the fact that at the time of miscarriage many women and some men turn to their mothers and fathers for comfort. (I limit the number of men who seek comfort because, as will be shown in many of the stories contained here, men often wrongly feel that the trauma is not their own. We are often depended upon for comfort and much less often considered the object of comforting, as if our involvement had ended with conception.) Understanding the generational/sexual link can help us understand why the turn toward home is instinctive and, probably, an effort to reestablish the generational line that has been broken. But there is another reason for understanding our biological link to our parents and the sequence it represents.

Alice and Joyce show us a situation in which lack of understanding of both basic sexuality and basic psychology kept mother and daughter from communicating the complexity of their feelings. Alice was unable to understand her own experience with miscarriage in part because she seems to have felt inhibited in any discussion that dealt with her own sexuality. If she had been more secure with her body and its functions and malfunctions she might have been better able to relate to her daughter's experience and, thus, able to offer the kind of comforting she herself had never been able to experience. The pain of the break in the biological chain was compounded by the break in the psychological ease with which one generation should be able to pass itself on to the next. Joyce, for her part a product of a generation that was encouraged to separate itself from its parents emotionally, wanted comforting in an area that had no foundation for an emotional exchange. Interestingly, both volunteered to me that they had never felt closer to each other than when the secret of Alice's hidden miscarriage was finally revealed.

Yet, even in relationships that are not strangled by emotional withdrawal, an incomplete understanding of generational linking can cause pain. My wife and I discovered this when we had our own miscarriage, and it took us several years to sort out what had happened.

My wife and her mother have the kind of relationship

most people only wish they could have with their parents. Because Eloise, my mother-in-law, has always been frank and honest about both her strengths and her weaknesses and has been open to changes in the dynamics of the mother/ daughter bond, Sam, my wife, has grown to value her as a close friend without ever losing respect for her as a parent. Sam has always been able to share both her joys and her frustrations with her mother freely and fully, with a sure knowledge that Eloise would join in both the good and the bad without judgment and with a steady and unqualified love. It was painful, then, for Sam to realize during her recovery from miscarriage that there was something wrong with what was happening between her and her mother.

Our miscarriage took place just before Christmas in 1981. We had already planned to spend the holiday in Raleigh with Sam's family. It is a pilgrimage we make every year with joy and excitement and great anticipation. The difference this year was that the day before the trip, Sam had had a D and C to remove the remains of our baby.

Eloise did all the right things. She was silent when Sam wanted to be quiet. She listened when Sam wanted to talk. She wept with Sam and she wept alone. She pampered and catered and held her daughter close when she needed it and kept her distance when she saw that Sam needed to be alone. She was as heartbroken as any mother could be and her sympathy and understanding were a much-needed salve for our hurt and confusion.

Unfortunately, for all the love and patience and sensitivity Eloise showed, there was still a place within Sam that remained uncomforted, cold and empty. It was not an obvious omission, and in the confusion of emotions and feelings that surrounded us like a jungle, it was hardly noticed. But it *was* noticed, and it continued to gnaw occasionally in the years that followed. It was not that Eloise had done anything wrong. Everything she had done had reinforced her love and concern and the extent of her empathic oneness with our trauma.

Yet something was missing—something Sam missed instinctively but did not know how to define. It was only when we began to discuss our experience again in the light of this book that we were able to identify what we think was the cause of Sam's minor but persistent disappointment.

Sometime in September or early October of 1981 Sam and I did two things. The more obvious of the two was that we brought into being a new life. Although it lasted only two short months, the life, the fetus, the baby was real and alive while it lasted. Which is why the other thing happened.

That product of our love—and our sexuality—turned us into *parents*. Before the conception we had been a close and loving couple. From that moment and forever after, we were the parents of a life. It was a temporary life, to be sure, but our parenthood did not end with the life of our child.

Eloise extended to Sam her love and her comfort, her heartbreak and her pain *as a parent to her child*. What she could not do was to recognize that Sam's grief was following the same sequence. Naturally, Sam was hurt both physically and emotionally. But instinctively Sam was grieving as much for her wasted offspring as for her own personal anguish. It was that space, that extension, that part of the sequence that was broken. And so that part of the pain went unacknowledged, untouched, and uncomforted.

Sam and her mother had always been open and frank about both emotions and bodies. Still, they stumbled. With Alice and Joyce the basic trauma of miscarriage was compounded by the stiffness of longstanding secrecy and the coolness generated by unprocessed pain. Alice, by a habit based on practiced ambivalence, deliberately disengaged herself from the sequence and the situation. Joyce felt that her mother was disengaging herself from Joyce as a person. That increased her hurt at a time when Joyce had all the hurt she could handle—both for herself and for her unacknowledged child.

Love and sex together are the emotional and physical

foundation of our passing from generation to generation. Perhaps through understanding the combination and frankly acknowledging the intricate network of both emotional and physical connections that constitute the generational sequence, we can begin to understand what is really happening when miscarriage seems to stop the sequence short. Perhaps grandmothers can learn to extend themselves a little further in the chain. Perhaps mothers can begin to understand some of the unnamed pain they are experiencing.

3

Jan

I wanted Jan to read drafts of some of the early chapters of this book. She knew nothing about the work I had been doing recently, but she is objective and honest. I thought she would be a good critic for some of the material I was preparing. When she answered the phone there was in her voice a quality that made me feel she had expected me to call but did not know it was me she expected. It was a combination of hesitancy and welcome that concerned me immediately. "Are you all right?" I asked. There was a pause.

"Walter, I had a miscarriage last week." We agreed to meet two days later.

I have said that miscarriage is frequent. I also said that its frequency is hidden by the fact that there is so little evidence of it. This came home to me so very clearly when I casually called Jan. I had not seen her in a few months. We have one of those friendships where we touch base every so often without having to be actively involved in the day-to-day of each other's lives.

I first met Jan about six months after Sam and I experienced our miscarriage. We were cast in a production of *Last of the Red Hot Lovers* at a small stock theater in New Jersey. It was my eighth production of the show. It was Jan's second or third. *Last of the Red Hot Lovers* is a war-horse of the small-theater circuit. With a cast of four and only one set it is inexpensive to produce and a solid favorite with audiences.

Barney, the middle-aged owner of a fish house, faces his midlife crisis by inviting three different women up to his mother's apartment while she is out. Each attempt at an affair fails, and the end of the play finds Barney on the phone trying to get his wife to join him. I was cast as Barney, and Jan was to play the first of my would-be conquests.

The company was put up in a rambling old house leased by the theater. It occupied a shady lot a couple of blocks from the theater itself and near enough to town that we could walk to most of the places we had to go. Cast houses are a unique form of accommodation. Half of the occupants are with the current show; half are with the show in rehearsal. The kitchens have a mismatched collection of dinnerware and utensils left by casts from shows long gone. Furniture consists mostly of props kept after plays have closed, so that a chair that blended harmoniously with the set of *Romantic Comedy* may sit in the living room and fight with the ideal sofa for *See How They Run*. It is an odd way to live, but one that actors have come to expect and, to a certain extent, enjoy.

Most people do not realize how long and hard an actor's work hours are. During rehearsals there is nothing but the script and the actors. When you are not in rehearsal there are lines to learn and moments to analyze. Focus, concentration, direction, dedication—this is all an actor knows during the preparation of a role. I can remember in 1967 mentioning the just-concluded Six Day War in Israel to a colleague who replied, "I didn't hear about it. I was in rehearsal." In that intense atmosphere friendships are forged quickly and well.

Jan and I had mutual friends. She had seen me recently in a show in the city. We found we shared a common faith. We quickly became buddies. One night soon after the show opened we were walking to the theater together and discussing intense personal crisis in the context of the characters we played. That led to my telling her about the miscarriage. It had been six months. I thought I was in control of the situation. I started the story confidently enough. Suddenly, in the middle of a sentence, in the middle of the block, unexpected and unwelcome, there was a rush through my body and I started sobbing violently. I was surprised and embarrassed and angry with myself and pained all at once. Jan, wisely and with compassion, neither judged nor counseled. She just stood there and felt hurt with me for a moment. I will always thank her for not *doing* anything.

During the run of the show Jan made one trip home to New York on a day off. She came back in love. She had met Tom and fallen in love with him in less than forty-eight hours. She was not naive enough to trust this first flush, and she did not mind being kidded about "lust at first sight." But she held to a strong suspicion that the relationship might just be a major one. The following year they were married.

We would run into each other from time to time and chat periodically on the phone. We worked on planning a project together, and we kept up with each other through people who knew us both.

The Jan I have known for nearly four years is a strong person. She came from a severely broken home. Her alcoholic father divorced both her alcoholic mother and the daughters who were to stay with her. The mother was more involved with her illness than with her children. Jan grew up with a sense that she was on her own. Acting became a way to be vulnerable in a place where the vulnerability could be controlled, as the rest of her life became controlled.

There has always been about Jan a sense that every move, every thought, every gesture was observed and dictated to. That is not to say that she is calculating or manipulative. Far from it. She is honest almost to a fault. She is sincere and warm and gracious and compassionate. But each of those qualities seems to come off the shelf carried by a deliberate hand. She is aware of this characterization, as she is aware of so much about herself. She admits to perfectionism. She also tolerates it.

Let me not give the impression that I find anything objectionable in Jan's self-possession. No. Rather I feel good in her presence, aware that no falseness or flattery will come from her or be tolerated in me. There is something liberating in that level of frankness between people.

The source of the honesty was once the shell of control Jan kept between herself and other people. If people's proximity could be assessed and assigned, then their power to hurt could be undercut and managed. Honesty, truth, basic reality became as important in distancing people as in establishing communication. In this unusual tension Jan was able to move through life neither icy nor vulnerable.

The source of Jan's composure changed as she came to know and depend on the power of her Christian faith. As she recognized and accepted the work of God in her life there was a subtle shifting. No longer were people kept out on purpose. Jan would now welcome them, but they had to be comfortable with that same honesty and truth and basic reality she had always carried. Those elements remained the same; only their origin changed. Jan became a person who could be counted on to be objective in an active search for truth, compassionate in an honest empathy with pain, and frank in a genuine concern for people. If there was any hardness about her it was a hardness you could lean on, not a hardness that would exclude you.

The Jan who walked into the tacky little coffee shop that early June morning was a softer Jan than I had ever seen. She looked tired, and the strength I had come to expect from her seemed thin and fragile. She still radiated with the energy I had always found attractive, but now the energy seemed to be seeking rather than giving. Over coffee and toasted bagels we talked, quietly and honestly.

She and Tom had been married two and a half years now.

She had waited through several relationships to find the man she would spend the rest of her life with. "We had a powerhouse of a courtship. And we've had a thoroughly life-changing marriage. In some ways good and in some ways . . . The first year of marriage was devastating. I didn't want to be that changed. I had no choice, but I hated that part of it. But we were a wonderful revelation to each other." Tom is a psychiatrist and a similarly devout Christian. His manner seems shy and deferential on first meeting. Later you realize that the quietness comes from conviction and determination, just the qualities that would be needed to share a molding process with someone as self-aware as Jan.

In the spring she had gone for a visit with her family in California. Jan's mother had died several years before, and with her death a lot of forgiveness and cleansing had taken place. Jan and her father, who is now a recovering alcoholic, had both grown up over the years and there was a great sense of reunion with him and with her sisters, both of whom have families. "It's interesting to see someone you grew up with have small children that look like you remember their mothers looking thirty years ago." Now there was a real family that Jan could relate to. Jan's father made the point that they just could not allow themselves to be separated. They were, after all, family.

Jan and Tom had thought about conceiving before, but neither had felt entirely ready to be parents. After the California visit Jan knew that she was ready. Tom agreed.

"My mother and my sisters were very fertile, and it never occurred to me that I wouldn't conceive immediately. I know myself biologically rather well, and I felt like this was the night and now was the time. We conceived first night out, and I just knew it. I had a kind of smugness about it." She paused a bit. "Yet I couldn't believe it. A level of me intellectually knew it and accepted it and began to revel in it, and another level of me—the mysterious level—said, 'This is the biggest thing that has ever happened to you and you're not *on to* it yet. You don't understand it. You don't accept it. You're not open to it.' It's something that the only real response to is submission. And I hadn't submitted to it totally yet."

In a couple of weeks Jan began to bleed. Just a little at first. It was a surprise. She used an 'at home' pregnancy test the next day, and the test was positive. She called her regular doctor. His advice seemed unsatisfactory: "You can't shake a good apple off the tree." With Tom there to handle any medical emergency, she called a midwife she knew, a very conservative caregiver with a sound medical backup. "She was concerned. She told me to get my butt into bed and stay there. Get out to pee and that was all. So from the very beginning I had a very quiet time. I was literally in bed."

Jan stopped for a moment and a curious thinness came into her voice. "I remember the first day, a friend came over to visit me. And I was lying in bed. I had laid out my wedding dress on the bed with me and I was holding the wrist—I was literally holding hands with my wedding dress. I got out every women's magazine and every cookbook and every item of domesticity around."

Her voice got stronger as she spoke of her faith. "I also began to face God, to turn myself toward Him and face Him. Because it was a position I was totally vulnerable in. I'm used to assuming some of the control. Now I began to accept the fact of how weak and helpless I was. I was shy. I was almost virginal in my response. I was awed. It was like the wedding night."

The waiter came to refill our cups, and Jan leaned back in the booth where we sat. Her wild black hair, which had always seemed so vibrant and alive, looked a bit limp. Her hands, which had always moved with surgical precision, seemed tired and defeated. I wanted to say or do something, but then I remembered her wise, silent response to me and just continued to listen.

"I went to a wonderful midwife. She is a wonderful caregiver in every respect. But she was very straight with me. From the very beginning she restricted my activities, she restricted my exercise, she restricted sexual expression. And she said, 'Your pregnancy is threatened.'

"At first I said, 'You mean it *might* be threatened.' But she said, 'No. It *is* threatened and you could be miscarrying right now.' After two weeks of my being in bed she took a blood test and she felt the pregnancy was sustained. Tom and I prayed twice a day. I prayed alone. I memorized the Magnificat. There was this mystery that every woman, including Mary, had accepted—this total lack of control." Now her voice grew thick and dark and her eyes began to redden and grow wet. "I realized that my baby, through this process, was telling me that I was a person submissive to a mercy and a majesty. The baby was ministering to *me*. The baby was telling me who I was.

"I was just beginning to understand it completely, when the midwife took a second blood test and she said, 'I want the doctor to see you immediately. Your hormone level has dropped considerably.' I had felt very woozy. I would feel like I was fainting. I just thought it was the pregnancy. Now I realize that it was the hormones dropping. But I also felt more like myself, too.

"Tom took the day off and went with me. It's the only time in my adult life that I have physically trembled. I was so frightened. And then the doctor gave us a good report. I looked, sounded, and felt pregnant. I could be having fibroids that were causing the bleeding. But I exhibited all the signs of pregnancy. He wanted to give me a sonogram just to back up what he was saying.

"We were elated. We went out celebrating. It was about four in the afternoon before we had a chance to eat and we got pizza. We ate *so much* pizza. And I was jovial and happy and I felt so good that I went to the sonogram by myself the next day."

I could tell what was coming—both by experience and

43

by the tension I felt in Jan. By now the sonogram stories had become familiar. So many of the victims I had interviewed had spoken of studying the glowing screen as the technician passed the scanner over their bellies. The images were strange and wonderful and confusing and, all too often, still.

"That was the worst," said Jan coldly. "I badgered the radiologist into telling me her findings. She was so terse, and at first she kept saying, 'The doctor will explain.' I knew the news wasn't good. And I told her, 'I know you're not my physician, and I'm not going to hold you accountable. But tell me what's going on!' And she said, 'At eight weeks we look for thus and so, and we just don't see it. There are signs of disintegration.' I said 'Level with me,' and she looked at me and said, 'This pregnancy isn't viable.'

"That night was the worst night for me. I kept wondering, Was I or wasn't I? I felt ripped off: Who had I been singing to? My first response was very selfish. I had given up an acting job for this pregnancy. I could have been out swimming all this time. Then I began to realize that this special person who had told me who I was maybe wasn't there. I had sworn that after I had the baby I would have a drink and Chinese food because those were the things I didn't want to have while I was pregnant. I came home and I had a drink. Then later at dinner I ordered Chinese food. And I remember thinking that this was really no consolation.

"The doctor said that it could be a mistake. He'd seen sonograms like that before that were wrong. He's a Catholic, and he wouldn't want to terminate anything that might be viable. So I just went into a dull holding pattern.

"On Monday, Memorial Day, we went to the Museum of Natural History. My husband loves dinosaurs. The place was crawling with children. And in that museum, in that dinosaur exhibit, I saw some little two-year-old number trotting across the floor holding his father's hand, and I knew that I wouldn't give Tom that this time. That was it for me. That was the end. We had to leave. That was when the depression set in. The next day I started to bleed and I called the doctor and he said wait for my husband and then get right to the hospital.

"I felt relief. I knew it was over. And I really felt great about going to the hospital. I knew that I wouldn't have a miscarriage in the supermarket. All those wonderful people in the hospital. They put you in bed and treat you like a princess. And I let them give me as many pills and as many shots as they wanted to keep me painless.

"When I woke up Tom was there. He's really a wonderful husband. And a great doctor. And my favorite human being. I felt totally cared for by him. In the hospital Tom and I were teasing each other. I was relieved. It was a crazy kind of punchiness. I had the same feeling when my mother died. I had the same humor making the funeral arrangements. It was just the relief that it was finally over."

We talked about the actor's habit of keeping a bit of perception free during even the most devastating crisis. It is that little bit of artist that watches and says, "Oh, so that's how that feels. File that one away for future use." Jan admitted to that. But then she said, "I got a job right away. That was a miracle. I went to the reading a week to the day after I got out of the hospital and I knew that I gave an audition that was at least sufficient and probably excellent. And it was a better role than the one I gave up for the pregnancy. And I knew I had done well and they knew it and we all knew it and we all went home knowing that they were going to hire me to do the role. Usually that is a marvelous experience for me. What it did this time was make it very clear to me that I would rather have a baby than do a play. It was like, 'So what.' "

When we talked, Jan was still very close to the event. She was still bruised and tender. She may yet find some solace in work, or in simply rediscovering the love of husband, friends, and family. The doctors have said that she and Tom will be able to try again. She is a person who has always managed her life and her art carefully, the clearly etched outlines of the characters she has played corresponding to the strict rule she has exerted over the progress of her personal life. Now she knows the overwhelming helplessness of being at the mercy of a situation that totally dominates, to which one wants to be submissive and over which one has no control. Such experiences diminish some people; they can make others grow. By defining our response to our own weakness we can, ironically, become stronger, wiser, and ultimately, more human.

I saw Jan and Tom a few nights later. She still looked drawn and tired. She and Tom seemed especially close, and he was particularly caring around her, although he, too, seemed tired and a bit fragile. They are still in the wounding phase. The pain is still fresh. Everything they encounter, every smile from a friend, every song on the radio, every prayer or touch or scent or movement is, in some way, dominated by their loss. This summer's sun will not shine on their baby. Their neighbor's cat will not amuse their baby. Their baby will never hear this favorite hymn or TV jingle or love song. And each phone call or note, each conversation, each gesture of friendship stabs with a special agony that seems to add to the proportions of the event instead of reducing it. Few things hurt more than accepting sympathy.

But the wounding will end, eventually. The healing will begin, eventually. And, eventually, they will go on to live the rest of their lives. If they are like most other couples they will find that they are changed. They will have recognized the wounding phase for what it is and will have allowed it to give way to the healing time. If they are like most couples, they will then find themselves different, stronger, and more mature human beings. It usually happens that way—eventually.

4

Events, Feelings, and
the Psychology of Pain

S he was ugly. There is no other word. She was not just plain. Her looks were not just severe. She was ugly. Her nose was like a scythe cutting her head in half and extending well beyond her face like the profile line of some primitive idol. Her cheek bones were like knife blades lodged in the sides of her head. Her eyes were too small and set too deep in their sockets. Her lips were too thin and pulled tight against her bony jaw. Her lumpy body did not walk; it fell from one place to another in pieces. And her horsey cackle could cut through thunder and still be irritating. And yet, there was about her a sweetness and generosity of spirit more giving and open than almost anyone I have ever known. She seemed far more at ease with herself than most beauties I have encountered. Perhaps she had come to see herself realistically. Perhaps she knew better than anyone else her limitations and had chosen to forgive herself for them and simply be her own person.

No. Not her own. For she had given herself to him and in that love she felt a security that allowed her to stand proudly, her too-small head held high above her dumpy body.

He was not a visual prize, either, though people did not cut their eyes furtively at him as they passed in the street. Rather, he had a sturdy peasant build that gave him the distinct countenance of the unextraordinary. This was intriguing since he was one of the most decidedly extraordinary men I have ever met.

He was a painter, an actor, a director, a writer, a poet, a philosopher, and a failure. He was talented in all of these areas. If you asked him he would tell you just how talented he was. If you did not ask him he would tell you anyway. That seemed to be the basis for his talent for failure. His ego knew no bounds. He could enumerate in precise detail just what was wrong with every successful film, play, or television show. He could point out the weaknesses and blind spots of every successful painter, actor, director, writer, poet, and philosopher working.

As a painter he could create light satiric cartoons of cheerful wit and little consequence. He saw himself as a social critic. As an actor he created bizarre characters that were memorable. He saw himself as a great romantic tragedian. In print he was interminable. He saw himself as misunderstood. There was nothing realistic about him.

There was also nothing boring. At least not for her. She worshipped him, and when friends got fed up she would quickly say, "You have to make allowances. He's so talented. He doesn't realize how he goes on and on."

I met them when I was in my teens. During my twenties I followed the pattern of most of the people who tried to be close to them. He had given me some valuable career advice and help early on. Later I realized he was trying to run my life as he tried to run everything around him. I had grown older and less fascinated by negative banter. What had once seemed sparkling wit and a colorful array of talents grew thin and revealed itself as self-destructive self-deception. What had seemed the magnetic pull of the unique became self-serving egotism that sapped the time and energy of anyone standing too close. He had a way of giving unsolicited advice and then being angered if it was not followed to the letter. He seemed to assume that he was the final authority on every subject and that to disobey his command was a kind

of disloyalty. I distanced myself from him, finally only re-
gretting loss of contact with her. We did not drift apart. We
found ourselves rowing in opposite directions.

Over the years I had picked up bits and pieces of their
story. They met working on a play. She had a fine voice and
a wonderful way with character roles. Behind the mask of
makeup and costume she was at her most personable and,
oddly, her most attractive. He was going through a messy
divorce. They became friends and lovers. They did not plan
to marry. Then she got pregnant. They got married. She had
a miscarriage soon after the wedding. Soon after the first
miscarriage she had another. This one damaged her in some
way. She would have no children. The only times I ever saw
either of them vulnerable were when mention was made of
miscarriage or of children.

I cannot forget the many kindnesses they both showed
me over the years. The part of me that wants to be critical
must set aside the vivid humor and the thorough enjoyment
of good food, jokes, wine, music. They were among the first
adults who treated me, a teenager, as an equal. It was later,
when the sharing of their respect became a form of manipulation, that I had to break with them both. When I realized
that he was running both my career and my life, I balked.
What I finally recognized was that every conversation, no
matter whether it was about my career or a world event or
about a play or film we had seen together, ended with a
lengthy lecture about what he thought, what he knew was
wrong in the situation, and what he would do differently.
He was the one and only center of his own universe.

I remember a night when he was going on and on about
the fact that some people just should not have children because they did this wrong and they did that wrong. He was
endlessly generous with his opinions. Usually, when he got
off on one of his flights of indignation she was the only one
who could or would tell him to shut up and change the
subject. This night he was uninterrupted as he went from

what was wrong with children to what was wrong with parents and back again. His diatribe took on the character of a defense against his own lack of success at becoming a parent. His one-sided argument eventually began to suggest that if he were allowed to be a father he would know just what to do and when. Slowly the energy, the warmth, the very person drained from her. Quietly she went pale and hollow and eventually she slipped out of the room and into a private hell where pain was a constant and insensitivity was a sentence passed on her for the crime of not being beautiful.

There are two things in operation as I tell this story. One is, I hope, a brutally objective honesty about the nature of these two people and my experience with them. I have not been polite. I could have called her "not very attractive" and him, simply "difficult to get along with." Instead I have tried to be as frank and vivid as possible in offering a realistic portrait of them. I have not tried to be kind; I have tried only to be accurate.

On the other hand, I recognize in these harsh words my own feelings of disappointment, betrayal, and frustration with a friendship gone sour and with a situation over which I could have no control except to leave it. There is still pain in my words. Pain and anger and even, perhaps, a bit of hatred.

The important thing here is that by being honest with myself, both about the true nature of the people I have described and about my feelings toward them, the pain, the disappointment, the sense of betrayal, and the frustration are now in my words on paper, not in my heart or my mind. By being objective and realistic about what I will call *the problem*, and by being honest and open about *my feelings* about the problem, I have defused the situation, robbing it of the power to hurt me further. Do I still judge, pity, hate? Probably. But the energy I expend on that situation and the degree to which the use of that energy limits my present life have been greatly reduced by my being frank about the situation itself and open about my feelings toward it.

Miscarriage is a situation, like many others in our lives, over which we have no control. And we certainly cannot dictate in advance our feelings about a given event or person. Feelings come to us automatically and unbidden. What we *can* do is to be realistic about what happens to us and honest about our reactions to it.

This is not easy, particularly in the case of traumatic and painful events and people. Negative feelings are rigid and hard-edged. They are compact and forceful and unyielding. There is a self-satisfying crunch to the taste of hate and anger, a fulfilling wholeness in the feel of pain. These are not found in the giving of love, the sharing of kindness, the offering of forgiveness. But pain, depression, and anger are exhausting and sap every available ounce of energy. Healing, love, gentleness, these tend to energize and lighten our load. This is not just a philosophical argument. There is current medical research that suggests that the stimulation of the nerves and muscles that form a smile activate both the adrenal glands, which increase our energy and stamina, and the brain centers that release the biochemical material that registers in our systems as pleasure, whereas the neuromuscular activity that creates a frown has just the opposite effect.

What this means is that we have a choice. We can hold on to our pain, our anger, and our frustration and dwell within that thick dark place where our sensitivities are constantly bruised and our feelings are constantly negative. Or we can try to release our pain, let go of our guilt and our anger and try to work our way back to joy. That is never easy, as most of the stories in this book, including my own, will show. But it is possible. And it is desirable. And our attitude toward trauma has a great deal to do with how that journey back takes place.

The first baby I really remember was born to a family who lived across the street. We had moved to a small town in Virginia and we were renting the house we lived in while our new house was being built. I was in the third grade.

Our two families were not close. We shared a party-line telephone but I do not remember any conflicts there. There was just a style difference between our two families. I would say that we were simpler, and from the distance of some thirty years, they seemed to live a fancier life-style. Both houses were small matchbox affairs, square and divided into two tiny bedrooms in the back and a kitchen and living room in front. At the time the houses seemed comfortable, but looking back from adulthood I guess they must have been cramped and styleless. Perhaps that is why the lady across the street decorated with such unrelenting aggression. As I remember it, she had put ruffles and braid on everything. There were sculptured lampshades. There were fringed pillows. There were flounced curtains inside brocade draperies inside valances with scalloped edges. Her husband was a dump-truck driver.

Her daughter was a year or two older than I. She was blond and round and always wore dresses, even to play. And the dresses had ruffles and lace and rickrack and buttons. Her hair was always put up in ringlets falling from the very top of her head in a style known as "Little Miss Sunbeam" after the little girl on the Sunbeam bread loaf. I do not remember her name. We were not exactly close. It is just that there was a limited number of children in the neighborhood so we played with anyone we could find.

The mother got fatter and fatter and there was some talk about a baby. I was eight. One day the round blond girl came over to say that she had a new baby brother and he had almost all his fingers and toes but not quite and he was beautiful anyway. If I wanted she would show him to me. The offer was too good to pass up.

She took me in through the kitchen since the front door—

only a few feet away—was reserved for guests and, as a child, I did not qualify. We passed through the flamboyant living room and into the back of the house. From my perspective it was hard at first to tell what I was looking at. There were pillows and drapes and ribbons and puffs of fabric. There was a bed and on it lay a baby. "See," said the round blond girl. She held up one of the tiny hands, and two or three of the fingers stopped short just after leaving the palm. "There's one gone on the other side, too," she said, and sure enough there was a stump where one would have expected to find a finger. "Isn't he beautiful?" cooed the girl.

From time to time over the years I have wondered what ever happened to that little boy. He must be past thirty now. Surely he compensated for his handicap in some way. He may have children of his own today. We moved into our new house in another part of town soon after he was born, and I never heard of him or his older sister again.

The thing that stays with me, even today, is the contrast between that attitude that would try to turn even a matchbox house on a rough clay hill in a small town in rural Virginia into a fancy palace appointed to enhance the lives of a princess and a prince, and the reality of a handicapped boy born to a man who drove a dump truck. How flexible love can be. How happy the little round blond girl sounded when she said, "Isn't he beautiful?"

Our feelings and emotions are as complex, and as real, as the pain and grief that causes them. When they become too hard to handle it is often wise to seek professional help.

Jaqueline Lapa is a psychotherapist in private practice. Her training comes from a variety of counseling approaches and is aimed at helping her clients get in touch with the reality of their situations. When dealing with the pain of grief she points to several steps she takes that should help the healing process.

She acknowledges the value of peer counseling groups and of reading some of the literature on grief, including the writings of Elisabeth Kübler-Ross, who insists that grief is a healthy and proper emotion that will heal itself unaided if the sufferer will allow the grief process to do its work. When problems arise, however, there may be the need for outside intervention such as the one-to-one counseling that constitutes most of Jackie Lapa's work.

The first thing she tries to do is establish a safe space for the client to feel at ease in. This involves finding out what the pain is about and understanding for herself the grief that is causing the pain. "I can't hide behind a professional manner. I have to be real about the pain. I have to feel it too."

Once this initial phase has created a basis for a relationship she tries to help clients be open to their pain. "I think it's important not to block the experience of the pain. To be really open to it. It's much more painful to resist it than to fully experience it. Cry, scream, whatever!" She says that this can, in some ways, burn the pain out. "But," she warns, "there are a lot of mechanisms in each of us that don't want to do that."

She sees some clients who get settled into the role of victim. "There is a lot of secondary gain from being a victim. People feel sorry for you, you don't have to feel responsible for what you're doing and feeling. There's a lot of payoff for that role." As a counselor her role, then, becomes to challenge that. "I just can't buy into that. I have to let them know that they'll feel a lot better when they can take responsibility for how they feel." She maintains that in the process of fully realizing the pain, "Wisdom comes in—understanding—a peace about it. And that's the way to transcend it."

While she is working with clients who are experiencing the pain of grief she will often try to get them to step outside themselves, to let a part of them be objective observers focusing on how the body is reacting, how the breathing is affected, what is really happening. By doing that clients can begin to understand the objective reality of their situation and establish a meaning for the cause of the grief, to clean up any unfinished business, to grow as people.

Jackie Lapa knows this territory well. She has been around grief all her life. Her parents and her sister survived the Nazi death camps in Poland in the time of the persecution of the Jews during World War II.

Her parents set two very different examples for Jackie. Her father was never quite able to transcend what he had witnessed. His attitude remained dark even after he had settled what remained of his family in America. For nearly twenty years he struggled with the horror he had known. Finally, when Jackie was eighteen, he committed suicide. He had found no way to displace his pain or put it in perspective. Grief and depression consumed him, and life became a burden he was no longer able to bear.

Jackie's mother, on the other hand, faced life with a glowing goodwill and optimism that remained strong and uplifting all during the fourteen years she battled cancer. "I don't know if it's a particularly Jewish thing or not," says Jackie. "She seemed to have this attitude of 'pick yourself up and keep going.' "

The contrast between her two parents' attitudes may have had an influence on Jackie's early interest in psychology. Her mother's positive outlook was certainly a resource when Jackie suffered her own miscarriage during the third month of her first pregnancy.

Jackie and Richard had been together for seven and a half years, three and a half as man and wife. Richard did not really want children. He had made that clear. Jackie did and had made her position equally clear. The conflict was severe enough to threaten their marriage. But when Jackie became pregnant Richard grudgingly accepted the idea of parenting.

As Jackie told me the story a rather strange quality came into her voice. One moment she was forceful, determined to make me understand; a moment later her voice would withdraw as if she was not sure I believed her. But she continued, deciding finally to let the story speak for itself.

She was in a session as a client with another therapist. Like many mental-health professionals Jackie periodically enhances her own skills in this way. The object of this exercise was to allow images to form that would reflect any current conflicts in her own mind. Gradually she became aware of the presence of a being there with her. She took it to be the spirit of the child she had just learned she was carrying. The being let her know that it had two purposes. One was for Richard, to help him resolve the conflict he felt over the issue of having children. Jackie's issue had to do with abandonment. At the time she did not know just what the image of the being was all about. Later, during the pain of grief, she would recall the image and ascribe a very clear meaning to what it had told her.

She continued her work and her enthusiasm for her pregnancy in the face of Richard's resigned but still joyless attitude. She put aside the being and established a regular schedule of visits with her doctor. During the second month he told her to bring her husband with her the next time she came. There should be an audible heartbeat by then, and perhaps that would help Richard join in her elation. Richard agreed to go, and on the afternoon of the appointment he actually seemed to be looking forward to hearing his child. The doctor checked out Jackie and applied several instruments to her abdomen. But he never offered to let her listen to anything, and when the examination was over and she and Richard were sitting across the desk from him, he said that he wanted her to go that afternoon for a sonogram to check the health of the pregnancy. He was casual and composed, but Jackie and Richard both felt the seriousness of the situation and by the time they left the office Jackie was in tears.

Something in both of them was crumbling. Joy had carried

Jackie around on its shoulders like a heroic athlete. Suddenly she felt very alone, very lost, very . . . well . . . very *abandoned*. Richard, on the other hand, was experiencing a kind of clarity that all their arguments, all of her words and all of his resistance, had not allowed. For the first time he felt the depth of her desire to be a mother demonstrated in her fear and passion. Ironically, in grief Richard found himself changed, his wall of resistance fallen and his attitude open, for the very first time, to the possibility of welcoming parenthood. Later, in the change in Richard, Jackie would find the first small steps to her own healing.

The pregnancy was over, and in the months that followed Jackie felt the whole range of emotions, fears, guilts, and horrors that nearly every woman, and man, goes through following miscarriage. The characterization she uses is very telling: "As a woman," says Jackie today with particular clarity, "I really felt very unacceptable."

During that time the memory of the being who had come to bring Richard resolution and to focus Jackie on abandonment came back to her time and again. Soon she found herself at the edge of a spiritual precipice. She had tried to be a realist, firmly grounded in fact and objective cause and effect. She had often had odd feelings and experiences of a spiritual nature. Thoughts and images would crowd into her mind, but she would reject them, telling herself that her imagination was too active for a modern person in a scientific, technological society. Now she was not at all sure what the ground rules for existence were. "Finally I said to God, or Nature or the Universe or whatever, if you'll just let me get through a normal healthy pregnancy and have a normal healthy baby I'll be open to whatever that spiritual dimension is."

As she talks about it today it is clear that Jackie has changed. The two children that she and Richard joyfully parent have filled out her life and opened her to a range of spiritual dimensions she would not, could not, have known before.

And when clients come to her with the pain of grief she has a compassion and understanding that is true and real and open. She has been there. She knows.

There is a lovely moment in a play called *Teahouse of the August Moon*. Sakini, the warm, gentle, and charming Okinawan interpreter for the U.S. occupation forces during World War II, has just given the audience a short and delightful history of the various invaders who have conquered his people. "Not easy to learn," he says. "Sometimes painful. But pain makes man think. Thought makes man wise. Wisdom makes life endurable." And sometimes the wisdom that comes from understanding the reality of our own pain makes life even more than that.

5

William and Janet and the Actress

F irst, let us talk about William and Janet. You might recognize William if you saw him. You might not know his name, though, because he is one of those actors who works all the time, makes lots of money, and yet has never had a popular hit on television. People in the entertainment business know him. His face has helped sell shampoo and cars and radios and washing machines. Yet his name would not ring a bell to most of the audiences he has played for both on film and on stage. He is a working actor, not a star. He will probably always be a working actor and he will probably always live well. If he has had to compromise his early ambition to do great things and to make great art, he has, at the same time, been compensated in many ways for the concessions he has made over the years. One of those compensations has been the continuing love of his wife, Janet.

Janet writes. She has a dozen published books and many dozens of articles to her credit. They are not the novels she dreamed of writing. They are not always the daring exposés she had hoped to have published in major magazines. But her career has been fruitful and prosperous and Janet and William have had a life filled with tastes of all the benefits money and success can bring. Still, to them the greatest benefit has been parenting their two children, David and Diane. There would have been a third child, but it died before it was born.

David was just a year and a half old; Diane would not be born for two more years. It was Christmas time. They were supposed to be on vacation. Janet was three and a half months pregnant.

It had been a rough couple of years for the couple. Before David their life had been so simple. They were night people. Their friends were night people. William's schedule usually had him working in the theater in those days. Broadway audiences saw him play lots of nice medium-sized roles in lots of nice mildly successful plays. Janet would work at her desk from late afternoon until William got home at midnight. Or she would meet him after the performance and they would bar-hop with friends until the wee hours. They would fall into bed at dawn, sleep until noon, shop together or museum together or make love together all afternoon, and start work again as the sun went down. It was an active and delightful life, and the financial rewards were mounting. They had moved into an expansive apartment with a river view. They had bought a weekend retreat in the mountains north of the city. There were nice antiques to furnish their homes and nice clothes to wear to social events and nice people to know and sit up half the night talking with. Then David was born and things started to be not so nice.

David spent most of his first year crying. He had feeding problems and he had colic and he had rashes and he seemed to never sleep. And because he never slept, neither did Janet. Neither did she work. Neither could she meet William for a drink after his show was over or jump into bed with him whenever she felt like it—and she was too tired from being up all the time with David to feel like it very often. William did what he could. But he had to work to support his growing family. He started spending more time auditioning for commercials and less time discussing the art of the theater. He started taking small, well-paid roles in television rather than challenging roles in the theater that fed his ego but did not put as much food on the table.

By the time David started to calm down a bit—he was well past one now—the couple was exhausted and isolated and frustrated and nearly estranged from each other. Janet was pregnant again and they were not sure what the added burden of another child would do to their lives and their marriage. Their life was no longer active, it was reactive. Every change, every disappointment, every cry in the middle of the night took so much out of them both that they had no time to move forward. It was all they could do to hold on just where they were.

When William suggested a Christmas vacation Janet agreed as much out of habit as out of desire for a respite. If someone else would make the decisions and the plans she would go. She had no more decisions or plans in her. William got his mother to come to the city to take care of David, and the two tired people made their way to the airport.

Janet had felt a bit bad even before they left. But, in her condition, it had been so long since she had really felt good that she could not know that this bad feeling was something special. They arrived in the hot sticky island of Jamaica, went directly to their air-conditioned hotel room, and Janet slept for twenty hours. When she woke up she was spotting. The problem did not subside. Meals were brought to their room, but Janet could not eat. She could hardly get up. Forty-eight hours later the couple was again in the airport, waiting for a flight back to New York. They had not left their room in three days.

When their flight was called William put out his hand to help Janet up from the wooden bench where she sat. She started to rise. Then, suddenly, she was on the hard linoleum floor, unconscious. An English doctor was now beside them. He had been at the airport to meet a patient who was coming in from the States. He said he had called for an ambulance and offered William the choice between the municipal hospital or his private clinic. "We're used to dealing with pregnant women," he said with a slight smile. It hit William clearly that the man ran an abortion mill.

The municipal hospital was like something out of a bad movie. The open pavilion was the remains of a World War II army barracks. The tropical architecture gave it a low roof and a platform floor. The walls were supposed to be screened, but the screening had rusted away in the humidity and great open patches allowed flies and other insects open air space and free access to the patients. There were about forty patients, in varying degrees of distress, all in the same large room. They were all women. There was only one telephone for the ward. Janet was only periodically conscious. William felt isolated and intimidated. If he ever had to play a character who was alone in every sense of the word he would now know how that felt.

Janet began hemorrhaging severely, and William looked around for help. One of the two nurses brought him a towel and a moderately clean bedpan and told him to try to collect anything that came out. She then returned to the desk where she and the other nurse were cutting stars and snowflakes out of the foil liners of empty cigarette packs to decorate the small Christmas tree.

Toward sunset, as the tropical sky took on the vivid colors of a clear hot evening, the only doctor available did a quick exam and said that everything looked clean and so Janet might not need a D and C. But another doctor would have to see her, and he would not be in until morning. No one offered them food. Visitors came to bring fruit and bread to some of the other patients. The water in the tap was warm and foul-tasting. Then a voodoo priestess set up shop at a nearby bed and began to chant. None of the other patients took much notice. All night William sat next to his wife. The chanting went on and on. Janet tried to sleep. William tried not to think.

He had not wanted this baby. (Years later he would describe the event thus: "That was the baby I killed by not wanting it." The statement was made as a dark jest, but it was made.) Their lives were in such turmoil. So much had already been given up. It was wonderful to have a son, but David was difficult to handle. Their standard of living required so much income. The effect of another baby right now would have been . . . what? William could not say. He was afraid. He was frustrated. He had to manage somehow. But all his usual reference points were gone. Here he sat in this nightmare. And still the witch woman sat keening in the corner.

Morning came and so did the other doctor. He determined that Janet would have to be scraped out. There was no question of scheduling an operating room. There was only one and there were only the uninterested nurses to assist. They brought a stretcher still caked with blood and grime from previous uses. William followed them. When the operating-room door swung open he looked inside and his stomach knotted. The room was filthy, littered with the leavings of who knows how many other procedures. There were blood stains on the floor and used bandages and dressings everywhere. Instruments were soaking in a sink, but there was no sterilizer in evidence. The wood plank walls of the chamber admitted light and dust and insects. William was sure that he would never see his wife alive again.

It was during those awful minutes while he waited outside that hall of horrors that William came to a realization. More than at any time before—when he had been entranced by her beauty, when he had been proud of her publishing success, when he had been lustful of her tender body, when he had been charmed by her lilting laugh—right now he knew that he loved his wife. More clearly than it would have been possible to know outside this threat, William understood what love was and how it completed him and made him whole. Here on the edge of death he fully knew what life was.

I have known such a moment of clarity. When our daughter Tucker—in this context I must call her our second child—was born, it was by a hasty caesarean section. The prenatal testing showed that she either had a cardiac problem or was standing on the cord. In either case, although she was not due for another month, the doctors felt they could treat her more successfully outside her mother.

The operation took place at about five-thirty in the afternoon. Because of the suspicion of heart problems and because she weighed only a bit over four and a half pounds, she was immediately whisked away to the neonatal intensive care unit, where she would spend the first fifteen days of her life.

Tucker was the immediate concern. I stayed with Sam in the operating room until they replaced the drugs in the tube in her back with drugs in the tube in her arm so that she could sleep while they repaired the foot-wide hole they had cut into her abdomen. Then I went upstairs to visit our daughter. There were telephone calls to make and doctors to talk to, and I ended up spending the entire evening at the hospital. It was after midnight when I made my last stop of the day back on the delivery floor. Sam was still in recovery, groggy and with a pale color that turned her usually olive complexion to a strange peach tone. I asked the nurse when she would be moved to a room on the maternity floor. "Not for a while," she said with a professionally evasive air. I must have looked quizzical, because she added, as if I could be objective about such information, "Her blood pressure has not come down since the surgery. It's still very high."

The information was like a slap. The possibility that anything could go wrong with Sam had never entered my mind. That she could be in danger, that she could, in fact, be damaged or die from childbirth, seemed like something out of very old fiction. In the dreary Fathers' Room on the second floor of the hospital, I was forced to really look at love for, perhaps, the first time.

The Chinese have a symbol—the yang and the yin—that embodies the balance between positive and negative, dark and light, male and female. It is a circle divided by an S-shaped curve. Where one side is full and round the other side is thin and tapered. Where the first side is small and weak, the other grows bold and powerful. I think love is like that. In the stillness of that awful little room I suddenly knew that without Sam there were holes in me. Without her there were spaces and crevices and openings that no activity or person could fill. Where I was dark she was light and where she was weak I was strong and where I was night she was day and where she was cool I was warm, with the full solidity of unity and wholeness. For better or for worse, in sickness and in health, in richness and in poverty, in lust and in frustration, in joy and in disappointment, we love. And if we are able to be fruitful and multiply, that offspring is the product of more than simple biology. That baby is the result of our attempt, successful or not, to complete the circle, to match the strong and the weak, the dark and the light, the laugh and the tear. And when the attempt fails—when a baby miscarries—the circle is shattered, the unity is broken, the wholeness is diminished. If we can find the pieces and put them back together, we can survive. If we can recognize the shapes of the holes in our lives and fix the pieces in their proper places, then we can fulfill the full potential of our love. That is the way it was designed.

It would be unfair not to tell you that Janet did survive and recover and a couple of years later Diane was born. Today, some fifteen years after the miscarriage, they still live with their river view, William still maintains a profitable career playing financially flattering parts, and Janet has a new book ready for the publisher. They are a couple wedded to each other by vows, by their shared progeny, by experience and lust and predisposition and history and humor and habit. Most of all, however, they are a couple wedded to each other by a real understanding of the fact that they want to be important in each other's lives.

It is easy for me to identify with William's sense of confusion, frustration, and ambivalence over the loss of the baby, and with his sudden and clear realization of his love for his wife. Both sets of feelings resonate off some of my own experience and echo the experiences of many of the men I have talked to. What is most difficult for me to imagine is the sense of physical isolation and helplessness inherent in having such a trauma take place so far outside our usual expectations of what medical care ought to be and in a place where so many of the trappings of our everyday life are distant and inaccessible. Death, any death, is hard enough to deal with under the most pristine, comfortable, and familiar of circumstances. Add a faraway setting, a cast of characters ranging from the threatening to the grotesque, and you have a script that theater critics would condemn as "unlikely melodrama." And yet, these things do happen. Which brings me to talk about the actress.

She was nearly fifty and neither attractive nor affluent. She had spent most of her life raising three daughters—alone since her husband walked out some years before. She was an actress, but her attitude was tentative and her resumé was thin. She took all the right classes, but they did little to add technique and confidence to her basically drab countenance on stage. Fortunately there are some wonderful roles written for a drab countenance, and the play we were both in had one.

I was just a few months past our own miscarriage. I had hesitated accepting this part since it would mean I would be away from Sam for a month and a half. She was still treading water emotionally and waiting out the long grief that had followed our own trauma. But she insisted I go to work. She

70

thought the time alone might do her good. She also pointed out that a change would be good for me. And work has always had a healing effect. The play was now three days away from opening.

It was Sunday morning, and we did not have a call until noon. The previous show had closed the night before, and the technicians had spent the night dismantling the old set and starting the process of installing the scenery for our show. The kitchen of the cast house where the company lived was bright and cheerful in the morning light. I had gotten up early to do some script work alone with quiet morning coffee. I did not expect to see anyone for hours.

She appeared about nine-thirty. Morning eyes were puffy and red, and she looked as if she had not slept at all. I was concerned. We had an important scene together, and yesterday's rehearsal had gone very badly. She had been progressing rather well up until that point. Even the morning run-through had had life and spark and timing. Then during lunch she had gotten a long-distance phone call. The afternoon rehearsal of the scene was a torment for everyone concerned. She had no concentration, she had no timing, she did not seem to know her lines. She disappeared before supper time, and now in the morning light she looked dreadful. My first instinct was to ascribe her look of disorder to embarrassment over her poor representation in yesterday's rehearsal. After a few groggy morning exchanges I offered to go over the scene with her. She said that would be helpful a little later and continued to steep her already deep brown tea.

"I hope you're not upset about yesterday." I said it gently, but it drew a startled look from her. "We all have had days like that," I ventured.

She blinked as if listening to another conversation and mumbled, "No. I'll be better today."

During the couple of weeks we had worked together I had not seen her so distracted. "Is it something else?" I asked. She nodded. Part of her resisted clarifying whatever this thing was; part of her clearly ached to open up. I was worried now. I had charged in thinking something ordinary had interrupted the professional progress of our work together. I was suddenly aware that whatever the problem was, it had nothing to do with the play.

"Someone I know was in an accident," she said slowly, as if each word came out of a separate package and had to be unwrapped before it could be used.

"Bad?" It was feeble, but it was all I could manage. I assumed the worst and expected her to say so.

"Yes," was all that came back.

I felt like I had been walking along for some way and only dimly realized that quite a while before I had passed through a doorway. Now it was suddenly clear that I was deep inside this thing. "Was it one of your daughters?" I was horrified that I was now irrevocably a participant in something so intimate. I looked at her hollow eyes. "Was she . . ." I could not bring myself to say the word.

In the flood of tears and sobs that followed the bits and pieces of the story came out. Several months before, her middle daughter had left home to "find herself." She was nineteen, unemployed, and rebellious. She had checked in every few weeks and had called just a few days before her mother left the city to do this play. She was on her way to Hawaii with a friend she had met while waitressing in Seattle. The youngest girl, seventeen, had been planning to spend the summer in a job-training program. The day after rehearsals began she called her mother to say she was going to hitchhike across the country and join her sister in the middle of the ocean. Yesterday the Maui police had called with the news that the nineteen-year-old had been on the back of a motorcycle when a drunk driver careened into the bike. The boy driving the bike had lost an arm; the girl had, quite literally, lost her head.

I am glad I was there to help release the tension that had

been building in this pitifully isolated and helpless woman. She was so alone, and the full impact of the event would clearly not hit her for some time to come. As word got out the women in the company were able to trade off being available. We all became more understanding. She got through the opening and the rest of the run, and by the time we closed she was even having a little fun with the part. She had abandoned any thought of leaving when the police told her it had taken three days to reach her, the accident was long over, and the body had been readied for burial on the authority of the girl's friend from Seattle. She eventually caught up with her youngest somewhere in Texas and she had turned around and was headed back home. The grieving and healing that was yet to go on in this shattered family was awesome to contemplate.

Yet, my personal reaction was grateful. Several days later I realized that for months I had been carrying only two thoughts: work and grief. Now I had added sympathy. And the sympathy I felt was having an effect on my own personal grief. It was not that our tragedy was any less painful or wrenching or lasting in its effect on us. It was just that in the face of this outlandish set of circumstances I was able to put some of my pain into perspective. However awful our loss had been, I was able to see it was not experienced without the comfort of friends and family nearby. It was answered with love and hope and prayer and tenderness and patience, and it just was not as bad as some of the things that happen to other people. It was bad enough, but it was not this bad.

I tell these two stories to offer the same perspective to those who are trying to heal. It is an old and clichéd saying that 'I cried for shoes until I saw a man who had no feet.' Perhaps the bizarre stories will not lessen our immediate pain. But they can help the long pain settle more quickly.

Because at the heart of the cliché is a truth: There is always someone with a more appalling, more ironic, more frustrating or depressing or shattering tale to tell than our own. That may not help at the moment of crisis. If allowed, it may help some down the road. And, perhaps, it will give us the space in our lives to love a little more.

6

Doctors and Reality

F irst Dad's legs started to go. He complained of cramps when he walked more than a few feet at a time. Two bypass operations did little to help. His feet remained cold and purple. His kidneys began to fail, then his liver. He had already developed diabetes and quickly ran through the stages of oral medication so that he had to learn to inject himself daily with insulin. When his lungs started to fill regularly with fluid and press on his heart, the term *congestive heart failure* entered our vocabulary. My father is seventy-four.

Ironically, through most of it he has been able to joke and talk about current events and share his love and concern for our family. It was only recently that we discovered that he did not know where he was or what year it was or that his mother, who died thirty-five years ago, was not coming to visit this afternoon. When I finally talked to his neurologist he explained that Dad's brain was deteriorating rapidly and things would go from bad to worse. "Frankly, Mr. Williamson," he said gruffly, "the best thing your father could do right now is *die*."

It was a startling thing to hear. When I tell friends about it they are shocked and angered. I am no longer. Because of that blunt conversation I have not had a moment of false hope. I have not wasted any energy playing "What if?" The doctor was honest. My father is going to die, and if he does not do it soon we will be faced with the heartache of watching him deteriorate to a vegetative state in which body and mind rot relentlessly before our eyes. That does not diminish the love and pain we have shared in the past or change our disappointment at missing what we had hoped for in the future. But the doctor's frankness has made it possible for me to accept the primary reality that puts all the other realities into perspective.

I speak of primary reality because we spend much of our time and energy on a level of secondary reality. Everything from paved streets to air conditioners keeps us from a direct relationship with the reality of nature. Three-minute film clips on TV become substitutes for whole wars. Muzak and greeting cards become substitutes for experienced emotions. Drugs and alcohol become substitutes for physical experience. Our society encourages us to dwell at a safe remove from the reality of our daily lives. But when the air conditioner breaks down, the heat seems unnatural. When the television is on the blink, the quiet and isolation seem unreal. And when we are faced with the death of a parent—or a child—if we have never come to terms with the reality of death, death itself seems unnatural, unreal, and unacceptable.

When my wife's grandmother had a heart attack in her eighty-fifth year she was hospitalized and attached to a monitoring device that beeped and flashed with each beat of her damaged heart. Sitting in her room we became aware of the fact that we were paying more attention to the machine than to Mama Perry. She was there before us, unconscious but real. Yet our attention was fixed on the beeps and flashes. *They* seemed more an indication of her life than the reality of her ancient chest rising and falling under the pale sheets of the hospital bed. We somehow found it easier to deal with the secondary reality of the machine than with the primary reality of the woman. The machine would not live or die. The machine would not feel or give pain. Dealing with the fact that the machine might stop beeping was easier than

78

dealing with the fact that Mama Perry might stop living. Secondary reality is attractive to us all because we instinctively know that it does not count. That is why we cling to it even when primary reality is available.

Crisis disallows secondary reality. Crisis makes us face life and death directly with no negotiation or manipulation to soften the vividness of the experience, for secondary reality is polite while primary reality is simply true. For most of us it is a wrenching event to be thrust into a situation that actually goes beyond success and failure and touches on the bare fact of life and the bare fact of death. Usually, the score-keeper, the official, the usher at the event is the doctor.

When Sam, my wife, missed her period and suspected she was pregnant, the first thing she did was call the doctor. When she told me about it one of the first things out of my mouth was, "What did the doctor say?" When she began to bleed our first response was to call the doctor. In addition to being stewards of our ongoing health, doctors, in a very real way, are our monitors of life and death. Perhaps that is why we instinctively invest them with an almost priestly power over our lives and the lives of those we love. Perhaps that is why they sometimes assume that position on their own.

But doctors are human, too. We look to them for knowledge and for objectivity and for a dispassionate professionalism in the face of events that destroy our own well-tuned composure. Then we sometimes turn around and complain that they seem cool in the face of our grief. I talked to one doctor who claims that what we sometimes see as insensitivity is actually trained into medical students. "That first year," he said "they stick you in a room with a dead body and tell you to start cutting. No one helps you through the emotions. It's sink or swim." This doctor had gotten permission to develop a sensitivity workshop with some of the residents at the hospital where he teaches. After a few sessions the Chief of Service came to him, furious. "What the hell are you doing?" he shouted. "One of my best residents broke down crying in front of a patient with cancer. Another one has quit altogether. This sensitivity nonsense has got to stop!" Yet this doctor also told me of a call from a patient who was very dissatisfied with the attitude of a specialist he had sent her to. "I said, 'I'm sorry, but the fact is his mother had just died that morning and he probably wasn't himself,' and she said to me, 'Well, that's not my concern!' "

In *Look Homeward Angel* Thomas Wolfe puts one of the most beautiful evocations of the human condition ever written into the mouth of Dr. McGuire. "Oh, we're a flash of fire," says the old medical man. "A heart, a brain, a spirit. We're also nine cents' worth of lime and iron we can't get back." It is important to remember that that description applies also to doctors.

My friend Jane was very helpful in fixing the role of the doctor in the miscarriage process, as well as in understanding the doctor-patient relationship. Like most of the victims I have talked to, she had experienced good doctors and bad ones. Her former doctor had responded to her symptoms too late to save her first pregnancy. Now with a new doctor and a new pregnancy she had begun to dilate in the fifth month. She was on a routine visit to that doctor when he noticed that she was showing signs of opening. He immediately moved her into surgery and sewed up the mouth of her cervix. She would remain on her back in the hospital for the next two months in the hope that the baby would stay in place. From her hospital bed she was delighted to talk about her history and her perception of what a good doctor ought to be.

At first she had been with a doctor who was very patronizing. When she and her husband decided to have a child she realized that if this man was patronizing about simple infections and routine gynecology, he would ride roughshod over her when it came to a pregnancy. She changed to a woman doctor with some sense of relief. She was very confident in the new doctor's medical ability for the five years of their relationship. Ironically, she found the woman to be less delicate than any of the men doctors she had been examined by, but their rapport was good and Jane soon felt very much at ease. It was the group practice that finally drove Jane away. The morning of her miscarriage her regular doctor was involved with another case. The senior doctor in the practice put Jane off and told her to wait. "He didn't know my case. He acted as if I was just another hysterical woman. The more he tried to calm me over the phone the more frustrated I became." Finally, it was too late.

One of the hardest things Jane ever had to do was change doctors. "At that point it's almost like a divorce," she said. "You imagine the old doctor will think of you as an ungrateful wretch or respond in anger like an ex-spouse. This is someone you have trusted with your *life*. This is someone you have shared your fears and your safety with. But it's important to remember that you're not looking for a friend. You're talking about hiring someone. This is a business relationship. You began it; you can terminate it."

Jane had heard about Dr. Ming-Neng Yeh at Columbia Presbyterian Hospital. Several people she knew had found him remarkably competent and caring. And he has an impressive rate of success with high-risk pregnancies. Jane enumerated the things she likes about him. "He is very dry and he doesn't volunteer as much information as I might like. But if you ask him he will tell you. After all, if you're old enough to be a mama, you're old enough to get all the facts. He doesn't diminish your concerns, but he doesn't hold out false hope. He is conservative in his expectations, and he is extraordinarily cautious. He allows plenty of time for questions. And that time is sitting down in the office after you're dressed, not while you're still trying to get your feet out of the stirrups. He seems to recognize that physical well-being is only part of the relationship. I think one of the most important things about him is his sense of peace. You really feel that the health and safety of your baby is his first priority."

Jane told me about an enthusiastic resident giving her a checkup a couple of days after she was admitted. He asked if Dr. Yeh had discussed a new drug procedure with her. He said he would talk to him about it. Jane later asked Dr. Yeh about the resident and the procedure. "He was so . . . so *compassionate* is the only word. It was too early for the procedure. But Dr. Yeh didn't dismiss the idea. He was open to it and to the enthusiasm of the resident. I think that *compassion* is the thing I like most about him."

On the way to meet with Dr. Yeh I thought back over my own history with doctors. My mother was trained as a nurse. I grew up in a household that regarded doctors with both reverential awe and realistic scorn. At various times in her career Mother had watched doctors destroy themselves with "alcohol and wild women." She had also watched miracles of wisdom and skill in operating rooms and in farmhouse beds. I can remember with great pleasure hot summer nights when the rest of the house was still. Mother and I would drink the last of the lemonade and she would tell her stories. I heard most of them many times, but it did not matter. All through my childhood I soaked up both the human weaknesses and the superhuman power of the medical profession.

There was the time the victims of a road accident were brought into the emergency room. A truckload of chickens had collided with a truckload of eggs. Wounds were filled with eggshells and feathers and dung and splinters. There was the time a doctor had asked her to go out to an isolated farm to assist him. When they got there there was no electricity and, in the middle of the night, she had helped him perform an appendectomy by lamplight. There was also the doctor who was missing when his own son was brought into the hospital. In front of his wife someone had called the home of a certain nurse where he was known to spend his off-hours.

In more recent years Sam and I have often compared notes

on the many doctors we have met and dealt with during the eight years of fertility testing that led first to our miscarriage and later, joyfully, to the birth of our daughter. On the one hand, there was our first specialist. He was a hearty but humorless man who approached examination with a kind of energetic objectivity that made each of us in turn feel more like a specimen than a person. Objectively I knew that I functioned well on a mechanical level. But subjectively, I feel sure that none but the most brazen and dramatically endowed could have his penis *evaluated* without at least a flutter of paranoia.

For Sam, the process was even more involved. She, too, was poked and prodded. Then she was injected with dye and gas and stretched and examined and x-rayed. Private parts are just that—private. Yet male genitalia are evident and visible any time the man is naked in a communal shower or on a liberal beach. A woman's working parts are hidden from sight even when the woman is undressed. This must surely contribute to the tradition that expects a woman to be more concerned with modesty than a man. And it must surely make the sense of violation, even for valid medical reasons, more extreme when relative strangers go exploring.

On the other hand, there was Dr. Reyniak, who saw us through the miscarriage and carried us on to our second, successful, pregnancy. Sam came home from her first visit smiling. She liked him personally and professionally. But she was also struck by something in the way he worked that had nothing to do with medicine. "He was dressed in a blazer and slacks," she said, "and when he came in to do the pelvic he didn't change into a lab coat. He just washed his hands and proceded with the exam." I did not understand why that should be so shocking until she explained that this was the first time she had been to a doctor who did not put that white coat between himself and his patient. Somehow, unconsciously, the white coat had always been a signal that something dirty was going to happen that would stain or soil the doctor's clothes. Dr. Reyniak's blazer became an important symbol of the confidence and comfort he inspired in us.

When I got to the hospital where Dr. Yeh maintains his office I was struck by the ways in which medicine has changed over the years. At the entrance to the building there were signs for half a dozen clinics, treatment centers, and research labs. There were security guards and metal detectors and directions to meetings and conferences and symposia and classes. On the side of the building, however, over the old entrance that is no longer used, there are only two words: *Babies Hospital.*

Like any large teaching hospital, this one was a hive of activity. In the lobby there was a very pregnant woman in distress being attended to by a gray uniform, a green uniform, a white uniform, and a very anxious husband. Hundreds of doctors, nurses, and patients filled the halls and elevators. Snatches of conversation overheard included only occasional syllables I could understand. "Her da-da-da-cardio-da-da went into da-da and we had to do a da-da-da-bypass in order to get her calcium-da-da back up to da-da. Larry did it last night."

By contrast, Dr. Yeh's office was quiet and calm. His patience was evident as we talked through some of the standard information available in most consumer texts about the causes and classifications of miscarriage. He mentioned some of the more usual conditions: incompetent cervix (the condition that my friend Jane suffered from), improper gene linkage, tubular pregnancy. He underlined the fact that there is considerable diversity in the degrees of both physical and emotional response. One woman may bleed dangerously; another may notice no more than a heavy menstrual period. One couple may be traumatized profoundly; another may quietly absorb the loss and continue to function freely and well. He was careful to make few generalities. I got the distinct impression that he prefers to treat each case as a unique condition, relying on umbrella terms only in deference to my lay status. He did not burden me with more jargon than was necessary about his own area of success, working with hormonal causes of miscarriage. He was also honest to say that many of the triggers of miscarriage are not understood.

He defined the timing used to determine the difference between miscarriage (up to twenty weeks) and prematurity/stillbirth (after twenty-four weeks), and acknowledged the gray area in the time frame. He was gentle but exact as he outlined the various combinations of time and circumstance in which the fetus is either alive or already dead at the time the body begins to reject or accidentally eject it. The word he used was *abortion,* and it was a stumbling block for me. But Dr. Yeh made it clear that the word simply means the stopping of a pregnancy.

Dr. Yeh did not reveal any new information during our hour together. Most of what he described I had encountered in one form or another before. But in him, as Sam and I had experienced in our association with Dr. Reyniak, I recognized those qualities his patients had lauded: Absolute medical authority coupled with absolute honesty about what the medical profession does and does not know and can and cannot do. Sincere compassion for the patient's situation coupled with respect for the patient as a person. An enthusiasm for the workings of nature and a degree of humility in the face of all the variations that nature permits.

When I asked Dr. Yeh why he got into the OB/GYN area he displayed just a trace of personal emotion. "In Taiwan, when I was in training," he said carefully, "I was assigned to a ward of terminal patients. There was very little we could do except make them comfortable. I knew right then that I wanted to be part of the beginning of life, not the end."

Perhaps that is what we all want.

7

Mary and Dave

I t was a mild June Friday and traffic and pedestrians along the avenue were starting to take on the extra energy of early summer. The gray chill of a particularly cold and difficult winter had been washed away by the spring rains and now the tender green of leaves just grown was deepening into the rich dark moss color of maturity. It would be a good summer after all.

Suddenly, people on the street looked up. The bells of St. Paul's church were pealing out with an unexpected and startling vigor. Those nearby looked at the front of the church expecting to see a wedding party emerging. But no bride or groom came down the steps. Could it be some national event or secondary holiday that had escaped their attention? Parishioners of St. Paul's, however, heard the bells and smiled, and many knelt in prayers of thanksgiving before rushing to their phones to confirm the good news.

In the church office the telephone began to ring. "A girl," the secretary said, time and time again. "Mary is fine. Dave is with her." A baby had been born. A little girl. Had the strollers in the street known that the simple birth of a healthy baby had initiated this surprising outpouring of rejoicing and concern they might have been puzzled. Had they known the whole story, however, they would more than likely have joined in the celebration.

Two days later, Father's Day Sunday, Dave Winters stood

in the pulpit of St. Paul's Church, faced the altar, crossed himself, and turned to the congregation. "Today might not have been a joyful day," he said, "but you risked that. You invested yourselves in this pregnancy and now you share our joy." He paused and looked around at the hundreds of faces staring up at him, many with tears in their eyes. "But," he went on, "there was the possibility that we could have lost it all, and then you would have had to share our grief. It was the *risk* that has touched us most." The congregation understood. They all knew the story. Mary had now had a baby. But on the way to this happy Sunday with its tears of joy Mary Winters had suffered seven miscarriages.

The first was a fairly neat event as miscarriages go. Dave was in seminary. Mary was in graduate school. They had been married about three years. Mary became pregnant. They went for a short vacation during which Mary was sick most of the time. When they got home they found that the pregnancy was over. Not an unusual event, even though it carried with it the usual grief and sense of failure. Naturally it was painful to face. But Dave and Mary were just beginning to learn about pain.

By the time Mary had carried her second pregnancy for three months she hoped that whatever had caused the first to end had been an aberration. They were living in the city now, and their doctor was part of a very well recommended and fashionable practice. When she started to spot she was upset and called the doctor's offices. Her regular doctor was not on the rotation that night, so she had to tell her story over the phone to a man she had never met. Apparently she sounded hysterical. In fact she was. But the doctor seemed to discount the degree of her pain and fear based on the fact that this was a hysterical woman he had never met—and what was he supposed to do over the phone?

Dave took her to the emergency room. They looked her over and sent her home. *Typical* was the word someone used. Mary's level of hysteria was not diminished. Nor was she calmed the next night when the hospital took the same attitude. Four nights in a row Dave and Mary went to the emergency room for help only to be turned away. Her doctors had no appointment time and each in rotation gave her platitudes over the phone.

On the fifth night she was in pain. The bleeding was heavier. They had been trying for days to get someone to help them. Suddenly, in the emergency room, Mary went into convulsions and a senior doctor was called in. As he examined her, the increasing urgency in his manner and in his instructions to the nurse frightened Dave. "She's bleeding internally," the doctor said. "My guess is this has been going on for quite some time." Dave wanted to scream.

"That's what we've been trying to tell you people for five days," he fired back. But the doctor was deeply involved in his work, and an angry husband was the last thing he had time for.

"Hold her down," was his only instruction to Dave as his whole arm seemed to disappear inside Mary. "We'll have to abort right now," said the doctor. "And if I can't get this bleeding stopped she may have to have a hysterectomy as well." There was no time to absorb the danger. Dave watched in horror as the medical team went into action. Now there were instruments and pumps and receptacles all around. Blood was everywhere. Mary was pale and only semiconscious. Frantically the doctor worked between her legs as red-stained gauze littered the floor and lumps of tissue were withdrawn and discarded. Somewhere in the back of Dave's mind the life of their second child was crying out for attention. But in front of him the life of his wife was in jeopardy. There would be time to grieve later.

Finally it was over. The nurses and orderlies began to clean up the mess, and the doctor stretched and took off his grotesquely smeared gloves. Dave, still holding Mary by the shoulders, watched for some sign of comfort or instruction or, perhaps, just an explanation. The doctor looked back

91

with an ironic twist at the corner of his mouth. "It's a shame," he said, "that we didn't get to this sooner. It wouldn't have been nearly as much trouble." And he turned and walked away.

Mary's own doctor was professionally sympathetic, but told them it was important to get pregnant again right away. Very little energy was wasted on understanding what had happened, and few words were used to comfort the couple.

As an assisting priest in his parish Dave was assigned some of the less convenient services to perform. A few days after the bloody night in the hospital it was his turn to offer the early morning Eucharist. It was a small service and sparsely attended. Dave stopped at the entrance to the chancel that morning and made a resolution. Between Dave and God it was decided that this regular ritual would stand for the funeral that was never offered for his son.

One of the glories of the Episcopal tradition is the liturgy that serves as a guide for every ritual in every season. This great poetic work has changed little in the hundreds of years since Henry VIII divorced the Church in England from the Church of Rome. Any Episcopalian can enter any Episcopal church anywhere in the country and know immediately where to join in the worship. This consistency is designed as a framework for prayer so that each phrase can have its own meaning for each participant, yet all are bound together by the common repetition of the basic words.

At one point in the service the celebrant holds his hands above the bread and wine and speaks the Words of Institution. On that morning, as he finished the Sanctus and lifted his hands into position over the chalice and paten Dave kept before him the image of the fetus he had seen so briefly in the emergency room. "For in the night in which he was betrayed . . ."—the word had an odd ring to it today. "He took bread and when he had given thanks, he brake it . . ."— brake, broke, broken. Promises, hopes, dreams had been broken. "This is my Body, which is given for you. Do this for the remembrance of me." Good-bye, dear son. I will remember you.

The doctor had told them to get pregnant right away. Yet sex was no longer free from a traumatic history. The second miscarriage had been so violent, so physical, that it carried a sense of rape with it, and Dave and Mary both felt an uneasy tension even as they sought the joy and comfort of each other's arms. Dave had not been an actual participant in the violation of his wife. But he had cooperated: He had signed the consent form. He had helped them hold her down. He had watched as those things had been done to her. Now as he approached his wife he felt that he was opening up the possibility of all that happening again.

Pregnancy number three seemed to be going well for a while. But as she neared three months Mary could not avoid a vague feeling of foreboding. This feeling was given clearer focus when, during a regular Friday visit, the doctor picked up his telephone and asked a sonographer to see her that afternoon. He did not tell Mary that he suspected the baby was dead. He did not tell her much of anything. Neither did the sonographer. He simply asked Mary to sit down in the crowded waiting room after the procedure was over. Mary's mind raced as she sat there among other women whose faces displayed varying degrees of hope and fear. Then the receptionist called her to the desk and handed her the telephone. Her doctor was on the line saying, "Well, this one's gone, too." Alone and exposed, Mary struggled with the storm of emotions that swirled about her. But the doctor was still talking. "About half the fetus formed as a grape-arbor mole— in little clusters of tissue—very unusual—we don't see it much except in Oriental women. I want you to come in on Monday for a biopsy." The word hit her like a fist.

"Biopsy? That could mean cancer."

The doctor was patronizing. "Well, let's not worry about

that yet. I'll see you on Monday. Have a nice weekend."

Mary spent the weekend with the distinct feeling that there was a bomb in her belly.

By Monday Mary was tense and exhausted. The doctor helped her little by telling her that the results of the biopsy would not be ready for four days. He also told her that he did not want to remove the fetus until her body started to reject it. Mary tried to remain calm, telling herself that there was nothing she could do until the test results were known. That did not help her sleep. That did not help her relax at home or face the days with anything other than a thick veil of anxiety.

Thursday morning the telephone rang. Mary picked it up with a mixed sense of excitement and dread. But the doctor tried to reassure her immediately. The biopsy showed no malignancy. Then he proceeded to review the situation. The malformed fetus was dead. The pregnancy was over. But again he said it would be dangerous to try to remove it before Mary's body started the spontaneous abortion process.

The news was essentially good. She did not have cancer. They would not remove her uterus. Why did she not feel any better? She rested her hand over her abdomen. "Who were you, little friend?" she thought. "What were you, and where have you gone?"

When the doctor called again late Thursday afternoon Mary was confused. He spoke quickly, like someone trying to clear up mistakes. He had changed his mind about removing the fetus. He wanted her to check into the hospital that night so that they could give her a D and C on Friday morning. Mary agreed, but wanted to ask questions. Had he not said that a D and C would be dangerous before she started to abort spontaneously? What was the rush? Wasn't the biopsy clear? The line had gone dead. Mary had agreed to check into the hospital. Once he got that commitment he was not interested in saying more.

Dave took Mary to the hospital Thursday night, and on Friday morning she was put under the anesthesia without ever seeing her physician. When she awoke in the quiet room she could recognize Dave's hand holding hers. She turned to him with a questioning look on her still groggy face. "Everything's fine," he said. "They cleaned you out and there's no sign of any cancer or damage. We're free to try again." Mary was still befuddled.

"But where is the doctor?" she begged. "Why did he want to rush so?"

Dave felt helpless, angry, frustrated. "He's on a plane for Switzerland. He went ahead and did your operation so that it wouldn't delay his ski trip."

The first decision they made after Mary got out of the hospital was to find a new doctor. At the suggestion of a friend who had experienced pregnancy problems they contacted an elderly doctor near Boston who had been researching problem pregnancies for nearly forty years. The doctor was himself suffering from leukemia. He agreed nonetheless to see them, and so began a series of visits, tests, and procedures that eventually gave them a clear understanding of what the problem was and what to do about it. During the process Mary was to experience five more miscarriages.

The testing in Boston finally showed a specific hormone deficiency that was treatable. The prescription involved both injections and total bed rest. Because Mary's body processes that hormone at an abnormal rate, even moderate everyday activity would use up the injected supplement. If Mary expected to carry a baby to term she would have to arrange to remain absolutely bedridden for the entire pregnancy. Once this understanding had been reached Dave and Mary decided to take a break. They had been involved in failed pregnancies, medical testing, and grief for more than five solid years. Now that they knew what they would have to do they decided to take a year or two for themselves. In a very real sense their lives had become a function of conception. They felt they deserved a little time for just the two of them.

Before Dave and Mary committed themselves to resume their efforts to have a child it was important that they establish a relationship with a doctor in whom they could feel confidence. "I wanted someone who, if I called in the middle of the night with a pain or a problem, would take it seriously. Even if it did turn out to be nothing." Mary began to audition doctors. Her medical file was now several inches thick. She sent copies of it to several doctors asking them to read it before engaging in any discussion or examination. Several were patronizing. Several were too busy. One said to come in. When Mary arrived he said he wanted to examine her and run some tests before they talked. Mary was firm. "Either we discuss the file before we go any further or I walk," she said.

"Now, Mrs. Winters," said the doctor. "I think what you need is a fresh . . ." but Mary had picked up her file and was out the door.

From a parishioner who had experienced similar hormonal problems, Dave and Mary heard about Dr. Ming-Neng Yeh, who maintained a small practice connected to Columbia Presbyterian Hospital. Mary sent the file on ahead. Dr. Yeh called and asked them both to come in.

When they arrived they were hopeful but realistic. They were not medical experts. But they had become experts in their own condition, and they were now experienced enough to know exactly what they were looking for. When they were ushered into Dr. Yeh's office he stood up behind the desk where Mary's bulky file lay open, looking more like the contents of an entire drawer than the record of a simple effort to have a single baby. There was a long silence as the three people stood there. Then the doctor's head turned slightly to one side and his eyes grew soft and moist. "You've been through so much," he said with compassion and wonder and respect. Dr. Yeh became their new doctor.

In the early fall of 1982 Mary conceived a child. She and Dave were ready. Dr. Yeh was ready. The medical team at the hospital would be ready when the time came. But another element in this saga was also ready. This was a group of some fifty women from St. Paul's parish who committed themselves to help this child be born. Mary was required to stay in bed for the entire duration of the pregnancy.

Television, radio, books, and music could keep her occupied some of the time. But there were meals for her and for Dave. There was shopping and laundry and errands. There were the hundreds of details that mobility usually makes easy. Mary had no mobility. So keys to the apartment were left with several neighborhood businesses and with the doormen of several nearby buildings. Each day one of the ladies of St. Paul's would appear with lunch, mail, dry cleaning, whatever was required. They brought food and necessary services into Mary's life. But more than that they brought companionship and the knowledge that she was not alone. For eight months the Winters family numbered fifty-two. And a half.

Such a project does not happen by itself. This one was organized by a remarkable woman named Anne. She scheduled the visitors and sent Mary a weekly list of who was coming when. She herself came often and brought with her the good humor and friendship that Dave and Mary had appreciated in simpler times. In these more difficult times increased contact with her warmth and compassion were a major benefit of the experience.

It is a testament to the strength of this remarkable couple that they can tell their story today with a great directness and only an occasional trace of emotional vulnerability. "I use all the medical terms," said Mary as we sat over coffee in the peach-toned parlor of their rambling old suburban home. *"Fetus, spontaneous abortion, terminated.* I know if I really let myself think about them as children I couldn't live." Dave is now rector of his own small church some forty-five miles out of New York. The area gives them space and freedom to relax with their healthy two-year-old, Rose. Rose has her father's dark hair and acute angularity of movement. She has her mother's squarish features and forceful presence. Like any wanted child she is the center of their attention and the determining factor in the structure of their lives.

It was a bright March afternoon when we talked, and the green countryside was warming to the approach of spring. I had explained to them that I hoped telling their story and others like it would be of help to people dealing with the crisis that is miscarriage. They were anxious to be involved. And surely no one could have a better basis for involvement.

"You keep living for something in the future," said Dave. "And at some point you want to stop that and get on with your life. Our *identities* became 'those people who suffer miscarriages.' "

Mary is more ironic: "For a while our only friends were gay men. We just couldn't deal with couples who had children or could have children. Even single women were threatening because we presumed they were capable."

She talks about the fear generated by the extreme experiences of the second and third pregnancies. "When I got pregnant again I found myself walking to work in exactly the same pattern every day so that I would know every doorman and shopkeeper along the way—in case something happened."

Mary tries to be lighter and underline the funny aspects of the experiences. Take for instance, the party of dinner guests who were there the night Dave discovered Mary was pregnant before even she realized it. The couple had known that Mary became obsessive about tomatoes whenever she was pregnant. During one pregnancy she had made fresh manicotti every night for a week and loaded it with tomato

98

sauce. Now as they sat down to dinner, the guests stared at their plates with surprise. The china was piled high with sliced tomatoes and Mary was raving about how good they tasted. Suddenly Dave began to laugh. The guests looked in consternation from husband laughing to wife devouring tomatoes. Dave caught his breath enough to announce, "Mary's pregnant," and Mary was as startled as the guests until she looked around the table and realized that she had served each one a portion that could have fed a family of four. Then she began to laugh, too, and the following day her doctor confirmed that she was, indeed, pregnant again. A month later she lost that one, too.

"When it first started happening," she says, "we were in seminary and here were all these people who were supposed to be spiritual and they shunned us as if we had leprosy. They couldn't deal with the intimacy."

Dave had the same experience. He tried to beg off an assignment, but his rector insisted he conduct the funeral of a two-year-old child only a week after one of their losses. Objectively, it is obvious that either the older priest could not bring himself to do the service or could not summon up compassion for Dave's situation. Perhaps both were in operation. But that did not help Dave as he had to stand before the tiny coffin and speak prayers that were never pronounced formally for any of his dead children. "I think one of the hardest things," says Dave, "is to go through this whole death experience and there's nothing visible to mourn. It's so awful when it all gets taken away."

After Rose was born Mary had one more miscarriage. When it happened the couple decided not to try again. They had thought that having Rose might make it easier. It was different, but not easier. They do not want to face it again. Some might think that the more often it happens the less traumatic it becomes. The word from those who have been there is simple: "No."

Yet in our conversation I began to notice something interesting. When we talked of the miscarriages there was a precision and an objectivity that on the surface seemed almost cold. Both Mary and Dave, each in a different way, could recall specifics of the most traumatic times clearly and with little display of emotion. There was an ease about their remembering that placed the events at a distance and made the two seem more like narrators than participants. But when they talked of Rose the objectivity stopped and the whole level of energy and involvement changed. Mary had said earlier that she could not allow herself to think of the lost pregnancies as children. And Dave described with tempered emotion some of the same feelings of helplessness and frustration I had known once but at which he had become a practiced expert. Somehow the whole of their history was so overwhelming that to live actively within it would be too crushing a weight to carry even for people as strong and aware as Dave and Mary. Rose was another matter.

Mary speaks with wonder and appreciation of the daily treks of the women of St. Paul's to bring her food and friendship. And Dave warms markedly when he describes the spiritual climate into which Rose was born. He is realistic about the difference between the reality of parenting and the romantic image he held for so long before Rose was actually there to cry in the middle of the night or soil a favorite garment or break a treasured memento.

The difference becomes clearer as they take turns trying to occupy a tired and fretful Rose during the interview so that they can share the litany of their painful past with me. They *participate* in Rose's life. With all the other not-begun lives they remained observers. They experienced the physical and emotional assaults on body and mind. But they were kept from the one thing that parenting is supposed to be about: involvement with the *life* of your child. If living is about any one thing above all others it is certainly about sharing your life with the lives of others. Before any other accomplishment a successful life is marked by the degree to which the person living it is able to share, to be involved with, to participate in the lives of those around him or her. The horror of miscarriage goes far beyond the physical and emotional events suffered by the parents, no matter how extreme or how crippling. The real horror of miscarriage is that it slices through the line of love that should allow a parent to *participate* in the life of the not-born child.

Yet as I listen to the tape recording of our conversation another facet of this experience becomes clear to me. The one time Dave came near to tears was when he described the day of Rose's baptism. He speaks of the hundreds of people who were there to share the event with them and of the sense of spiritual and emotional community generated by her being brought before the altar to become a member of the greater church.

Let me warn you right now that what I am about to say will mean nothing to those people who firmly believe that we are born by accident of matter, live, die, and rot, period. To the rest of us, whether we believe in a formal expression of a specific relationship between creator and created or simply feel that there is some power "out there," perhaps this will have some meaning.

The sacrament of baptism is recognized by every Christian denomination. It is expressed in various ways, from the full immersion of some groups to the symbolic sprinkling known among many Protestants as *christening*. But the meaning is the same. By the act of baptism a covenant is established between God as creator and mankind as created. This covenant is as awesome in its implications as the covenants established with Abraham and Moses.

Our daughter, Tucker, was baptized in October 1983, almost two years to the day from the conception of our first miscarried child. The Episcopal liturgy provides an elaborate ceremonial whereby the congregation, and by extension, the whole Christian community, witnesses the event, renews its own baptismal vows, and prays for the spiritual growth of the newly baptized. But there is one moment in the service that is singular in its purpose and in its effect, and when it occurred for Rose I am sure that it had the same effect on Dave and Mary that it had on Sam and me when it happened for Tucker.

Tucker was dressed that day in a pure white gown that we borrowed from one of our godchildren. On her feet were tiny white satin slippers that Sam had worn at her own baptism and on her head was a cap that Sam's great grandmother had made for the baptism of Sam's grandmother. Family and friends had traveled hundreds of miles to be with us on this special day, and we had invested the event with as much tradition and earthly love as possible. Carol, our priest, had led the early part of the ceremony with that combination of devout faith and radiant goodwill that had endeared her to us in the bad times and made her an intimate part of the best times in our lives. Then she took Tucker into her arms and leaned over the water that a friend had brought from the River Jordan where Jesus was baptized by John the Baptist. She dipped into the bowl three times, washing Tucker's head, "In the name of The Father, and of The Son, and of The Holy Spirit." Then she said a prayer over our little girl.

What happened next, what follows in the ceremony, had a startling effect on me, even though I had read the words and stood as witness for many baptisms before. Carol placed her hand over Tucker's head and, with her thumb, made a cross on Tucker's forehead. Then she spoke, and her voice took on an intonation that was entirely priestly in that the priestly function includes speaking with the voice of God. She spoke for the first time to our child only, and the effect was of the creator of all that is speaking to this small created being. "Tucker," she said, "you are sealed by the Holy Spirit in Baptism and marked as Christ's own for ever. Amen."

What I felt but could not articulate then, and what engendered such strong memories in Dave as he talked about

Rose's baptism, was this: As parents we have enormous responsibility over the lives of our children. We join them at various times at various levels. We guide. We counsel. We discipline. We share. We hope. We enjoy our power and our involvement. But for those of us who believe in God—in whatever form—there is both a challenge and a comfort in the knowledge that, while our responsibility is clearly outlined by choice and tradition, ultimately we have no *authority* over the lives of our children. That authority remains with the creator and does not pass to those of us who, for all our love and concern, can neither create life nor take it away.

"If it matters," I said to Sam during the aftermath of our miscarriage, "God will explain all this to us one day." It was not much. But it contained a viewpoint that has become stronger in me every day I have lived. God is aware and in control. He is not removed. He is active. That said, our pain and grief are as real as the death of our children. Yet, that said, we are neither guilty of nor accountable for those deaths.

8

God, Priests, and Puppy Dogs

It was C. S. Lewis, the great British writer, who pointed out that we do not really know what we believe until what we *say* we believe becomes a matter of life and death. Our own priest describes it this way: You are hanging by a single limb at the edge of a cliff over a rocky drop that will surely kill you if you fall. You say, "God help me!" and the voice of God comes back: "Let go!" That is what faith is all about— letting go.

Our miscarriage took place over the course of a week. We were not in New York when it began so Sam's doctor had to do the best he could by phone. When she started spotting he told her to go to bed immediately. By the time he let her fly home to see him our baby was dead.

During that awful week we prayed a lot. Together and separately we asked God to either make everything all right or make us strong enough to face it if everything could not be all right. What He did was arrange for us to be totally dependent on Him. I believe that is how He wants it.

Someone once described the Bible as the record of God's attempts to offer mankind salvation and man's refusal to accept the offer. Although that description is facile, it contains a glimpse of how I believe God works. I believe that the creation of the world was a conscious creative act by an aware and compassionate being. I believe that there is a design and within that design a plan. I believe that God pays

107

attention to how that plan is unfolding. I do not believe that God usually goes around zapping people for doing things He does not approve of. (Usually. Read *Genesis* 19 about Sodom and Gomorrah.) Yet in order for man to know the creator, I believe the plan includes the possibility of pain and suffering. Each time a trauma occurs I believe He offers us the opportunity to either turn to the problem or turn to Him. Ultimately I believe that God wants us to turn all of our lives over to Him and allow Him to take both control of our actions and responsibility for our successes and failures. And I believe that God does not expect us to be entirely successful in that effort. If He did He would not have given us tears.

As a Christian I have specific beliefs about how that continuous offer of salvation has been presented. That is not what is important here. What is important is that the whole of Judeo-Christian teaching asks its students to trust God, let Him lead their lives; He then will act to make everything that happens work for His greater glory and their individual salvation.

It is necessary to understand this basic outline of existence in order to understand the nature of sin. Like most people, I grew up thinking that sin was doing bad things. It was not until relatively late in life that I came to understand that sin has very little to do with what we think of as good and bad. Sin is simply reaching that point where we can turn to God or turn to the problem and deciding to turn to the problem. Sin is the belief that we can control *anything* without the power and intervention of God. And we sin constantly. And God understands that and stands ready to forgive us and start again if we will only ask Him. The essence of all sin is estrangement from God.

"So?" you may find yourself asking. "What has this to do with the grief of miscarriage?" Just this: It was not until we went through it that I recognized just how much the grief of miscarriage feels like sin. There is the same sense of failure. There is the same sense of guilt. There is the anger of self-justification, which leads to the loneliness of estrangement. I was going to do something good. For some reason, which I cannot explain and do not know how to identify, I failed. Therefore I must have done it badly. I am guilty of doing something wrong, even though I do not know what I did wrong. Dammit! I did my best! How dare You or anyone tell me I am not in the right. No one understands me. No one cares. I am alone with my grief. (Notice all the *I*'s.)

It is so familiar. And so predictable. And so painful.

It is in crisis, be it miscarriage or some other trauma, that many people turn to God in the form of a priest or other clergyperson and ask, "Why did God make this happen?" Unfortunately, it is an entirely inappropriate question and will never get a satisfactory answer. God did not *make* this happen. He *let* it happen because it is within the same pattern of Nature that lets us *not* love Him.

I am no expert on the priestly function. In order to sort some of this out and put it into a professional perspective it seemed obvious that I should talk to a priest. I chose Fleming Rutledge.

She met me with an open hand and a smile and ushered me into her cozy office. She made coffee fresh from a tiny grinder and said again, as she had over the phone, "I really feel very uncomfortable about this. I've had very little experience with miscarriage. I don't know what I could say that you could use." She is slender and handsome and her black three-piece suit is a stylishly feminine version of the garb one might expect on a priest. But the bright red ribbon tie adds both color and sass to the ensemble and speaks of humor and joy under the cool professional façade. Fleming Rutledge is an ordained minister. She is also a wife and mother.

She has not had a miscarriage. The closest thing she can recall is the distressed birth of her younger daughter. For a week and a half the infant lay in the hospital. They did not know whether she would live or die. She did live and joined an older sister as part of the Rutledge family. But even today her mother's soft Southside Virginia accent tightens slightly as she describes the experience. The description occasions a question about the difference between the death of an infant and the death of a fetus. Her answer is direct: "When you have a visible living baby in front of you that you can look at, you are so sensible of the connection between you and it, whereas we've conditioned ourselves to think of fetuses as just tissue." On that basis she can understand the frustration felt by so many miscarriage victims. If the pregnancy was just tissue, why should it hurt so? If the pregnancy was, in fact, a person, why do so many people rush to dismiss it?

I ask about her approach to counseling someone in pain. What guidelines does she use? "I tend to resist the idea of guidelines." She smiles, and the smile is warm and genuine. "But I have certainly learned that there's no use talking to a person in pain unless you're willing to come alongside. So you become a listener in solidarity with the sufferer without necessarily having to go through the same experience yourself. You don't start talking about answers until you've shared the problem."

She fills my coffee mug and settles into the other armchair. She looks anxious and says again that she does not know what she can add to a discussion of miscarriage. I explain that I have not found anyone who seems to have a good answer to the problem. She accepts this and we go on.

I ask about the role of the clergy in crisis situations. She talks about finding the balance between practical psychological techniques of listening and expressing empathy and the role of the priest as a sort of theological spokesperson. "People don't come to a priest unless they expect to hear some 'God talk,' " she says. "But the only thing that can really make a connection is that solidarity, that 'coming alongside.' " She smiles with warmth and care and speaks of a friend, "a late Sixties-style priest. He would visit every day and listen forever. But he never prayed with the people. I don't even know that he was a man of prayer. That listening, that being there is wonderful, remarkable. But that's not the only function of a priest. They could have gone to a Jewish psychiatrist for that."

"Then what do you say," I ask, "to someone who has been told that it was God's will?" She shifts in her seat, and I can almost see her prepare for battle. "I think it's wrong to teach people that if you become a Christian everything will work out, and if you pray to God He will answer you, and if you ask Him for healing He will supply it. I think that's wrong. There's a lot of that teaching going around today, but I think it causes a great deal of anguish because people then think that if they're not healed, or if their child is not healed, then they have not had enough faith." She pauses. "So much of life is ambiguous. I was shocked to hear a man on one of those Christian radio shows talking about coming to terms with a child who was born deaf. He said that someone had pointed out Exodus 4 to him." She reaches for her Bible. "Here it is," she says, finding the place with the ease of familiarity. "'Who has made man's mouth? Who makes him dumb, or deaf, or seeing, or blind? Is it not I, the Lord?' " She lingers over the page a moment and then says, "I think if I were in pain and someone gave me that verse I would throw something at him." Her light laughter is clearly a prelude to something. "It's the old theological dilemma. If I say, 'God did this,' then I make Him a kind of monster. On the other hand, if I say, 'God did not do this,' I make Him an impotent bystander. There are some things that just have no answers. There are times we just have to fall silent."

We are both taken with the thought. After a moment she says, "I don't think we should ever take it for granted that people know what the content of the Christian faith is, no matter how long they've been going to church. We need to keep saying it over and over—whatever pain, whatever doubt,

whatever anguish, whatever despair you may be feeling—
God has not remained aloof from it. He has not looked down
on it from on high. He has himself entered into it. We believe
in the resurrection. But we are still here in sin and death.
The Christian life is one of hope for God's future, not one
of totally present fulfillment.

"And," she says, "there's always Psalm 88. That's the one
with no hope at all in it. I find that comforting somehow.
Scripture allows us to just shake our fist at God and say, 'I
hurt.' "

At home, after our talk, I looked up Psalm 88. As I read
the ancient words I was struck by the fact that pain has not
changed much in the thousands of years since it was written.

> O LORD, my God, my Savior,
>   by day and night I cry to you.
> Let my prayer enter into your presence;
>   incline your ear to my lamentation.
> For I am full of trouble;
>   my life is at the brink of the grave.
> I am counted among those who go down to the Pit;
>   I have become like one who has no strength;
> Lost among the dead,
>   like the slain who lie in the grave,
> Whom you remember no more,
>   for they are cut off from your hand.
> You have laid me in the depths of the Pit,
>   in the dark places, and in the abyss.
> Your anger weighs upon me heavily,
>   and all your great waves overwhelm me.
> You have put my friends far from me;
> you have made me to be abhorred by them;
>   I am in prison and cannot get free.
> My sight has failed me because of trouble;
> LORD, I have called upon you daily;
> I have stretched out my hands to you.
> Do you work wonders for the dead?
>   will those who have died stand up and give you
> thanks?
> Will your loving-kindness be declared in the grave?
>   your faithfulness in the land of destruction?

Will your wonders be known in the dark?
   or your righteousness in the country where all is
forgotten?
But as for me, O LORD, I cry to you for help;
   in the morning my prayer comes before you.
LORD, why have you rejected me?
   why have you hidden your face from me?
Ever since my youth, I have been wretched and at the
point of death;
   I have borne your terrors with a troubled mind.
Your blazing anger has swept over me;
   your terrors have destroyed me;
They surround me all day long like a flood;
   they encompass me on every side.
My friend and my neighbor you have put away from me,
   and darkness is my only companion.

I can remember sitting in a theater some three months or
so after our miscarriage. I was in rehearsal for a show. I was
off to the side studying my script while a scene I was not in
was being rehearsed. On stage the other actors and the director were busy building a warm comedic moment while
in the balcony some technicians were focusing lights. A conference was going on behind me about invitations for opening night. I could feel my chest and the muscles in my face
grow tense and hard and I was suddenly weeping great thick
tears that ran down my cheeks and stained the pages in front
of me. There was so much *life* going on, and I did not feel
like being part of life. I was part of death. I was alone and
frustrated and angry in my loneliness. I *resented* life. Then I
felt guilty about that resentment.

Guilt, in a spiritual sense, is the way in which God reminds
us that we are neither good nor powerful. In spite of attempts
in recent years by many religious bodies to deemphasize
guilt, it remains as part of our consciousness because it is a
basic component of the free will by which we disregard God.

There are plenty of studies of guilt available. Granted, most
have become deeply layered in dust in recent years. But the
research is there and I would strain your patience if I were

to try to cover that particular subject thoroughly. Rather, let me take one particular instance of guilt from my own experience and trace it through with you. It begins in a private dog pound.

We were looking at another puppy. The German shepherd seemed so frisky and energetic. We asked to see him out of the cage, and the man let us play with him on a table for a few minutes. We had just about decided on this aggressive one when I noticed Toby in the bottom enclosure. He looked up with his serious eyes and said quietly, "I'm here, too." I pointed him out to Sam as we put the shepherd back in his cage and we both knelt down to have a look. Toby brightened a bit and said, "You look like the ones I've been waiting for." He was tiny and quiet and the dark fur at his forehead came down into his shaggy gray face and formed perfect circles around each eye. He looked like he had glasses on and had just finished reading a serious tome.

We carried him home on the bus in a cardboard box. The ride and the excitement of having new parents at last were too much for him and he threw up sometime during the trip. When we got to our apartment we had to put him in the bathroom sink and give him his first bath. He was that small. He trembled as he said to me, "I hope you won't mind my saying this, but I'm not having a good time yet." He was six weeks old.

We dried him carefully and carried him back into the living room. We put him down in the middle of the floor and backed away. He blinked several times and looked around. Space! He sneezed once and said, "This is more like it!" He sniffed his way around the living room with growing speed and energy. Down the hall he ran and checked out each of the areas of his new domain. By now he was laughing, and when he got back to the center of the living-room floor he looked up with a smile, shouted, "Terrific!" and peed on the carpet. That was nearly fourteen years ago.

Toby died a few weeks ago. We had him put to sleep although we do not use that term around our two-year-old for fear it will keep her awake at night. Toby had been suffering with arthritis for several years. His knees had been operated on repeatedly and he could no longer lift his leg to relieve himself. He seemed to find that embarrassing and said so. He was nearly deaf, and he had become impatient with the baby. He could no longer walk very far without rest, and the two blocks of exercise and toilet we gave him three times a day were sometimes just too much. He would sit down in the middle of the sidewalk and look at me and say, "This isn't any fun anymore." A year ago he developed some tumors around his anus, and we had him castrated in order to slow the progress of the disease. But testing recently revealed a widespread cancer and the lumps in his armpits were growing at an alarming rate.

For twelve of his fourteen years Toby was our surrogate son. We did not dress him up or cook his food, but we thought of him as part of our little family. When everything fell apart, as it does periodically in everyone's life, Toby was a constant. He loved us mightily and forgave us everything. He always understood our problems and his counsel was consistent: "Dad . . . Dad, I love you." He was sensitive to our moods and knew when to leap up in joy and when to simply stretch out at the side of my chair and gently lay his head across my foot or stand beside the sofa and touch my hand with his nose. He liked to stay in touch and until he could no longer climb onto our bed he would sleep with his hips curled against my feet and his head against my wife's feet. We talked to him as to a child, and I would often call him son. He seemed to like that a lot.

Toby went everywhere with us. He loved to travel, and whenever we took down his suitcase and his traveling box he would leap and shout and play with obvious enthusiasm. He had flown more than many people we know. Summers he would fly with us on vacation or to whatever theater I was working in. At Christmas we made his airline reservations along with our own, and he would arrive at home with a large red bow, which he tossed with pride all through the holiday. His presence was always one of the best presents.

We have a storehouse of memories. Toby playing in the park with his friends Max and Cinnamon. Toby diving under the green sofa to fetch a wayward toy. Toby patroling the squirrels around our North Carolina house or chasing rabbits in the orchard. We have photographs of Toby by the fireplace and Toby gnawing on a bone. People would often say, "He just looks so much like Benji," and we would correct, "No. Benji looks like Toby." Toby would always say, "Thanks, Dad, for clearing that up."

We discussed Toby's death for several weeks before it came, but we had been aware for months that it was coming. Once the decision had been made it was a fairly efficient process. I called the doctor's office and told them that I was bringing him in and that I wanted this to be his last visit. They said they understood and that they would have all the forms ready when I arrived. I let him take as much time as he wanted as we walked the five blocks to the vet's. Once we turned the corner and got into the building I felt driven to get it over with as quickly as possible, but inside the actual office I sat down on the floor and gave him a last hug. I said a little prayer over him and handed his leash to the attendant. Then I sat down in the chair to sign his life away. A few minutes later they brought me back his leash and collar. It was all over.

I cried a lot. To hell with masculine role playing—I bawled my eyes out, there in the doctor's office and later with a friend who helped me to decompress. I did not want to go home and have the baby see me in that state. I was numb with pain and helpless with grief. And I stayed that way for days.

In the weeks that followed I tried to analyze my feelings. What I found fell into three distinct categories. There was realistic justification. Toby was dying of cancer. He was in pain and weak from the rapid spread of the disease. He was irritable and uncomfortable and he had no way to go off in the woods on his own or even to find a fully peaceful corner in our tiny New York apartment. Treatment would have been expensive, time consuming, and a crap shoot as to whether it would help or merely prolong the dying process. He could not hear well and he was beginning to leave food in his dish. His necessary walks would have been particularly difficult now that the snow season was beginning and he would have had to face salt on his feet and the cold in his arthritic joints. Objectively, realistically, and rationally, there is no question that letting him go was the right thing to do. He could not make that choice for himself. We had to, in kindness and concern, make it for him.

Against that objectivity there is the pain of loss and the cruel persistence of memory. Disposing of his medicines and putting away his leash called up visions that were clear and joyful up to the point at which we realized that they were all in the past. We still cannot bring ourselves to throw away his traveling case, and the sketch we had done of him at a street fair still hangs above the sofa on which he loved to curl up and nap. We walk through the door at the end of the day and miss hearing him say, "Oh, I'm so glad you're home." Returning from the bathroom in the dark of night I still tread carefully, expecting to encounter a hairy hip tucked next to the bed. There has been a death in our family. We are grieving and we miss him and the images of him will not go away soon and it hurts.

But there is another set of feelings more subtle and, in some ways, more painful. I have heard them suggested or admitted to in various hidden ways by several of the would-be parents I have talked to for this book, and the admissions echo off my own experience with both our miscarriage and with Toby's death. I am referring to a sense of relief. I am relieved that Toby no longer suffers. I am relieved that we no longer have his disposition hanging in front of us like an emotional waterfall we must drop over before the rest of our lives can begin. I am relieved that I no longer have to put on three coats and two scarves and take Toby out in the bitter skin-slicing cold at midnight to relieve himself into the salt-sprinkled snow. I am relieved that I no longer have to build schedules around the question of who will walk Toby or who will feed Toby or who will take care of the baby while I take Toby to the hospital if he collapses in the middle of the night.

When I talk to couples who have suffered miscarriage, some of these little reliefs, rationalizations, justifications come out whether they admit to them or not. They are inconsequential things like not having to give up a cherished apartment for a less charming one with two bedrooms, not having to change the style of vacations or evenings on the town, or even not having to wait any longer to know if this difficult pregnancy will last. They sound embarrassingly thin and selfish. But they are the only bright spots available in a landscape that has been benighted with the thick wet clouds of desperation, and they are clung to in the panicky fear that there will never be an end to this long dark night of pain. One victim was frank enough to describe it as the "flower planting" syndrome. "There for a while," she said, "I would dream that I was sitting on the edge of an earthen dam at the end of an enormous lake and I was planting flowers all along the edge of this dam to make it prettier, while beneath me the dam was collapsing and springing leaks and this disaster flood was coming and here I was trying to make it look as nice as possible." I knew immediately what she meant. I had felt it when our first baby miscarried. I had held tight to the surprise evidence that, after six years of fertility testing, we were not, after all, sterile. I tried vainly to see the miscarriage as a positive sign. And when Toby became so sick I actually sat down and wrote out a list of all the positive reasons for euthanasia. Later, I regretted both efforts. It was not that the relief was not legitimate or that the glimmers of solace were not genuine. It was that the event itself was so awful, so grotesque, so shattering that to find anything at all of comfort felt like a treacherous betrayal of the dead ones that was sickeningly self-serving and eternally unforgivable.

In my experience, and in particular at those times when I have grieved out of my assumed position as a parent, what God does is very simple. We try to carry the burden of responsibility and pain and guilt on our own. God offers to help us carry the burden. To our cry of, "LORD, why have you rejected me? Why have you hidden your face from me?" He answers, "I made you. I love you. *I forgive you.*" The extraordinary thing that happens is that God does what we wanted to do. God shows Himself to us as a parent.

9

Walter and Sam

"This is 'Sam' Perry," said Steve.

We were standing in front of the cafeteria at Louisburg College in North Carolina. Classes would start in another couple of days. It was 1966. Steve and I were theater students. Sam was president of the student government.

When we tell the story now Sam insists the first thing out of my mouth was a rude compliment concerning her chest. I cannot deny it because I do not remember a word of the conversation. What I do remember is suddenly being captivated by eyes that seemed to grow larger and deeper the longer I watched them. I remember golden hair swept smooth across her forehead and falling clean and straight toward her waist. And if my compliment was rude it could not have been totally unwelcome, for I remember that smile that opened her face and set her eyes and the air all around me vibrating with warmth and humor and light.

And then the conversation, whatever it had been, was over and Sam and her girlfriends were walking away. I turned to Steve.

"You know," I said, snapping my fingers, "it would take me about *that* much to fall in love with her." The truth was I already had.

There was little time for formal dating at Louisburg. We saw each other in the cafeteria and we walked to class together. We talked, we joked, she smiled, I basked.

There was a silly movie in town with Jerry Lewis and Connie Stevens setting up house on the moon. On the way back to Sam's dorm we sat for a while on the wall in front of the library. I told her that I was in love with her and that I wanted her to be the mother of my children. She sat quietly for a long time, just looking at me. Then her voice broke as she asked, in all seriousness, "Do you mean right now?"

There was no question in my mind. I was in love with Jean Simmons "Sam" Perry. I wanted her to be my wife and share my life. I wanted to go to sleep with her in the evening and wake up with her in the morning and through the day—and through the night—I wanted for us to do all the things that people who love do. Bewildered, she let me stay. But she would go quiet when I said again that I loved her and so I did not say it as often as I thought it.

At the Christmas dance she wore red velvet and the pink cymbidiums I had brought her. We danced, and laughed, but there were some unusual quiet moments as well. I let them pass. It got hot in the hall. We stepped outside for some air. Standing in the doorway with the light and the music on one side and the dark and quiet of the winter night on the other, Sam looked into my eyes. "I love you," she said, for the very first time. The flash in my head overpowered the flashbulb that went off near us. But later, going through pictures of the dance with Jeff, the school photographer, I found the portrait he happened to take of that moment. It shows the two people who at that particular time were the happiest two people on earth, and it hangs on our wall today.

A group of ancient oak trees surrounded the entrance to Merritt dorm. At night the lights of the dormitory porch would reach out onto the darkened campus. But the oaks stopped the light and made little coves of shadow, just large enough for a couple standing close, behind each tree. By common consent the couples who dated steadily adopted a tree as their own and as the curfew drew near each night the shadow coves would fill up with their regular customers.

At 10:28 Mrs. Bailey, the house mother, would step out of her apartment on the landing in front of the large front windows and begin making her way toward the front door. At 10:29, almost in unison, the sets of figures would emerge from the cozy dark of the trees and one figure from each set would head for the porch. At 10:30 Mrs. Bailey would turn the key in the lock and the evening was over. Watches were as important as textbooks at Louisburg in 1966.

As we stood in the dark by our tree that night I ran my finger along the edge of Sam's hair and down her jawline. She started to speak, but I put my finger to her lips. I had heard all I needed—all I wanted—to hear for this one wonderful night.

I believe in romance, and I pity people who insist that reality must consist of all rough edges and sharp corners. Love is real and it is not all rough and sharp, and people who want the beauty of beauty in their lives need only open their eyes to the beauty all around them. So it was that this beautiful moment had come. So it was that this particular beauty would stay here in this little rounded corner of time. I kissed Sam softly on each eye. Then Mrs. Bailey appeared in the front window. Then the ladies of the darkened trees gathered toward the porch. Then Mrs. Bailey locked the door and sealed the evening. Thank you, Mrs. Bailey.

We knew that marriage would not be easy. The vagaries of my profession were bound to create uncertainty and economic instability. But we were determined to try.

We were married on Saturday, June 14, 1969, at St. Thomas's Episcopal Church in Abingdon, Virginia. I was in rehearsals for a play at the Barter Theater. After a lovely small reception at the Martha Washington Inn we took off for a forty-eight-hour honeymoon near Hungry Mother State Park some thirty miles away. Sam was twenty-one. I was twenty-two.

At any given time more than 90 percent of the professional actors in this country are unemployed. I was employed under union acting contracts for 164 of the next 165 weeks. I was lucky and I knew it. But I had still not tackled the bastion that is New York.

So after a few years in regional theater we spent a few years in New York, where I continued to get work in regional theaters and had to leave Sam to cope in a city she did not like. When the opportunity came along for me to work in Fayetteville, North Carolina, as a resident arts consultant to the school system there we jumped at the chance. A year after our arrival we decided to get pregnant.

The first deliberately unguarded mating is a unique and memorable moment. Oh, how dramatic I was that night. Halfway through dinner it was clear that this was an "early to bed, late to sleep" evening. As we prepared to retire my wife reached for her little packet of contraceptive foam. With only a little less ceremony than is used to open the British Parliament I took it from her, walked across the room, and deposited it in the wastebasket. Even though we had been talking about it for weeks my wife was still awestruck.

"You're sure?" she asked with hope and love and fear mixed together on her lovely open features.

"I'm sure," I said. And that was that. Later I realized that the step we had taken had changed forever the character of our sex life. No longer was the act isolated. No longer was it only for the pleasure of sensual communication. Now it was a part of the continuity of life. Now it was a thing for all time.

I have already spoken of our frustration over the next six years as we tried to conceive a child. Let me only say that our continued failure was a major part of my decision to move us back to New York. If we were just going to be a couple, part of me reasoned, then we may as well risk everything for ourselves. I continued to get work out of town and took it with less and less reluctance. We continued to love each other and we continued to move through the maze of fertility tests that were consistent in their inability to help us.

When the Virginia Museum Theater called to ask me to play Marley's ghost and the Ghost of Christmas Present in *A Christmas Carol* in the winter of 1981, I accepted with pleasure. Sam and I made carefully detailed plans to connect in Raleigh with her family for Christmas day, and off I went to rehearsals in Richmond. I was surprised, then, when she called to say that she was flying down for the opening.

Opening night was a triumph for the production and for me personally. Sam arrived just before curtain time, but I did not see her until after the show. She was still in her dark-blue business suit, having had no time to change from office to plane to theater. The soft pink blouse and the pearls she wore dressed up the outfit, but they were no competition for the sparkle of her eyes and the warmth of her smile. Sam's eyes, which are deeper than most wells, and Sam's smile, which is broader and more cheerful than most sunlit valleys, would be suitable attire for meeting popes and presidents. These turned with full enthusiasm on me that night, I could not imagine myself more happy.

At the elegant party following the performance it seemed that everyone wanted to meet us. There were many comments about how like newlyweds we were followed by genuine surprise over the dozen-year duration of our marriage. Inevitably there was the question we had heard and danced around so often.

"Do you have children?"

"No. We're still practicing."

It had long been our standard answer, and it had lost some of its painful irony over the years of use. Nevertheless, "practice" was very much on my mind as we drove back to my room through the cold December air. Sam was smiling her secret smile, which usually indicates an anticipation of joy.

I was undressed and under the covers when Sam appeared wearing a gown I had not seen since our honeymoon. With trembling care she came to the side of the bed and placed a small wrapped package in my hand. To my questioning look she said only, "This is one opening-night gift you will never forget." Inside was a folded paper, and I knew what it said before it was even unfolded. There, in Sam's neat script, were words that spoke volumes: "You and I, by the grace of God, on or about August 8, 1982, are going to have a baby."

What followed involved no true sex act. But the level of joy and enthusiasm and energy and closeness would have been hardly distinguishable from the act that brought it about.

We laughed and planned and cried and prayed until deep into the night. Then we slept, and when I woke up the whole evening had a dreamlike tint in my memory. I looked at the nightstand and the precious note was still there. The sound from the bathroom told me that my lively pregnant wife was nearby. For a few moments I was alone with thoughts of my impending fatherhood. Then Sam appeared, and her face was almost as white as her gown. It was all she could do to speak, and when the words came they were halting and dry in her mouth.

"I've started bleeding."

We called her doctor in New York and, on his instructions, put her to bed in Richmond. We moved in a television and books and magazines and meals on trays. We talked with guarded enthusiasm about the baby. Sometimes I would come into the room and realize that Sam had been crying. Sometimes when I had to be out I would pull the car over to the side of the street and sit and weep for a while. Sometimes we would laugh and plan and pray together. Sometimes we would just sit quietly holding hands and hoping.

At the theater, news of the pregnancy got out and spread quickly. News of the trouble did not spread with equal speed.

Time and again well-meaning friends would stop me in the hall or stick their heads through my dressing-room door to say congratulations. For a moment I would have a flash of fully joyous reaction. Then an alarm would go off and I would find myself searching for tempering phrases. "Yes, it *looks like* we're going to have a baby." "We're *having a little trouble getting started*, but we *seem to be* pregnant." On the one hand I wanted to shout and sing the joy I felt with most of my being. On the other I knew I had to buffer my excitement to keep from being too disappointed if . . .

The bleeding continued but subsided somewhat, and after a week in Richmond the doctor in New York said it was all right to travel. He wanted to see Sam to get a better idea of what was going on. I wanted to travel with her, but she insisted I stay and do my work. Part of me was aching to be with her, to hold her hand, to give her courage. But another part of me was, quite frankly, relieved. I had vowed "in sickness and in health." I had not vowed to welcome the sickness part. If the news was good I would have wasted time and money and already rationed energy; if the news was bad, the selfish part of me said, there was little I could do except pillow the pain and try to absorb some of the sorrow. In less than two days she would be on a plane for her parents' home in North Carolina. We had already planned to spend the holiday there after my show closed. They could do as much as or more than I could. I did not want to be a coward, but everything was so confused with airline schedules and performances and calling friends long distance to make sure Sam was surrounded by all the comfort I could arrange via telephone.

Of course I had misjudged the difference my presence might have made. The whiplash plunge I had taken into and out of fatherhood had left me no perspective on either the problem itself or my capacity to help. In order to keep functioning I had become estranged from my own feelings. To an extent that I still feel uncomfortable with I had allowed my self-estrangement to distance me from the plight of my wife. If I had only known then . . .

When her call came the news was, of course, bad. I think I knew before she said it. "How are you?" I asked. There was a long interval before she spoke. Finally, the words came.

"The baby is dead." The sobbing that followed told me that she had not spoken those words aloud before. Speaking them was the most difficult and painful thing she had ever had to do.

It was a gray day in Richmond with a mist of rain and a cold lazy wind. As I drove through the streets the only levity I could muster was an ironic grimace at the fact that had I staged the event this is the kind of weather I would have ordered.

I found myself at a large church and asked if there was somewhere I could pray. The chancel was filled with pine trees and sheet-draped risers for the angels in their Christmas pageant, but I was directed to a side chapel that was dark and empty. Someone said he would turn on a light, but I hardly heard him. I felt my way into the area and in the gloom recognized the brass edges of a kneeler set in front of the brass fittings of a small altar. In the darkness I knelt and tried to ask God to sort out all the conflicting feelings.

There had been so little time to adjust to it all. The pregnancy was such a surprise after all those years. I had only had a few hours of unclouded anticipation before the bleeding had obscured the process and thrown me into an almost mechanical mode of dealing with the practicalities of being a helpful spouse. My performing duties at the theater continued eight times a week. Part of me was almost relieved that the wondering was over. Another part of me condemned myself for feeling any lightening of mood. Surely, I was not supposed to feel that way. The problem was that I did not know exactly what I was supposed to feel. There I was "planting flowers" and caught in the painful tug of guilt and relief.

As Christmas Present I had a scene with two children. After showing Old Scrooge the love and hope and faith and joy that exists all around him the ghost also shows him the faces of Ignorance and Want. I knew only that I was holding the two young actors particularly close these nights.

As I knelt there in the dark something like a bandage began to seal up the loose ends of my emotions and pack away my feelings in a pale, misty padding that would travel with me without being part of me for some time to come. In the terminology of Christian orthodoxy I had asked God to carry the weight for me and He had accepted the burden, for the time being. But while I was praying there, someone had turned the lights on around the small altar, and when I opened my eyes I realized that this side chapel was being used to store props for the Christmas pageant. There in front of me, but just out of reach, was a baby in a manger.

We got through the holidays. With as much grace as we could muster we smiled and chatted with friends who did not know, and we were brave and a bit vulnerable with friends who did. We opened our packages and made appropriate sounds of gratitude, and we tasted the rich food and made proper sounds of appreciation. When we were alone we touched and talked a bit. But we did not say too much and our touching was mostly to maintain contact while the storms of emotion and confusion, frustration and pain whirled around us. We did not understand. We were hurt. We did not know what to call the pain or why it hurt so much. After all, it was a disappointment and not a tragedy. Wasn't it?

We got back to New York and started to pick up the pieces of our regular life. I had several auditions that week and Sam went back into the routine of her work at the bank. We said what was necessary to get from morning to night. When our first weekend came we faced it with a cold distance that we neither wanted nor knew how to break. It was that Friday evening when I sat down next to her and waited for something to happen.

I do not know how it started or much about which of us said what. I do know that I asked her forgiveness for not being more present during the worst of the times. She understood. Then, as we peeled away the layers of defense that had piled up during the past several weeks, we got down to the place where Sam told me the details of her visit to the doctor. He had explained that the baby was dead and that she had two choices. She could wait until her body decided to expel the matter that made up the pregnancy or she could go ahead and let him do a D and C so that the physical trauma would be over. Slowly, between sobs, she guided me through the hell of that procedure.

There was the glass jar that collected the blood and tissue. There was the sympathetic expression on the face of the nurse. There was the sound of the vacuum pump. And there was the phrase that has haunted me ever since—the phrase that broke both our hearts again: "And then he sucked away what was left of the baby." Any objectivity I had been able to maintain vanished. At that moment I was, at last, able to participate in, to share, the horrible loneliness of that event. I stopped hating myself for not being there. I stopped being thankful it was over. I stopped trying to be helpful or brave or strong. I just sat there holding Sam and hurting.

I think that night marked the end of the wounding. What followed was the dreadfully slow process of healing. It was a strange and dangerous journey. At times it seemed it would never end. I remember us trying to comfort each other one night when we both found ourselves crying over a disposable-diaper commercial on television. Sam's red and tear-stained face turned to me and she asked, "Will we ever laugh again?" We knew we would. But at that moment laughter seemed years away.

10

. . . And After

Sam and I passed through the long winter and into spring in a kind of fog. We got from day to day with as much gentleness and concern for each other as we could find. Friends were faithful and mostly indulgent. Our work with the young people at our church was sometimes painful, but it helped keep us from withdrawing in self-protection from contact with children. I did a show Off Broadway and another on tour. I finished writing a play I had been working on. Sam joined a couple of committees at church. We coped. We continued. We survived.

By early summer the pain seemed to have passed. Most of the time we could function, do our work, meet and share with friends, worship, enjoy, and, yes, even laugh. But every now and then without warning we would turn a corner and run into a mother with a stroller, or see a news report about a sick child, and from somewhere deeply hidden would come an anguished flood of emotion. The times were not regular and they diminished in frequency. But they did not stop entirely and they have not to this day.

In August our doctor cautiously went through our history with us. For over seven years we had been trying to have a baby. We had been through every available test and procedure and we had had the one unsuccessful conception. He could not point to a reason, and his gentleness and concern tempered the frank statement that it did not look like we would have children. He was not about to say never. But he had done all he could do and we had certainly done our part. We seemed to fall into the small percentage of couples for whom there is no explanation for infertility. There are those who say that *cancer* is the most frightening word in the English language; *infertile* is the cruelest.

We went home that night and prayed together. We told God that we were putting our future in His hands. We had done all that we could do. If He intended us to have a child He would have to help. The ball, so to speak, was in His court. In October we were pregnant.

When we left the doctor's office we went to a coffee shop and sat down trembling with joy and love and excitement. We made a pact that we would enjoy every day, every hour of this pregnancy for as long as it lasted. In fact, it lasted until the following summer, when our daughter, Tucker Jennings Williamson, was born. I speak for both of us in saying that the days of that pregnancy were the happiest days of our life as a couple. Somehow every minute was precious, and we experienced it fully and with an appreciation that may not have been possible had we not known the alternatives.

I wish that I could say specifically what events or actions constituted the healing of our wounds. I am not even sure that they ever fully healed. As seems to happen with most victims, our born child now keeps us moving forward with such force that there is little time or energy to look back to our not-born one. It is not that we have forgotten. It is just that there is so little place now for remembering. Present joy and pain and work and sharing and the ongoing process of *living* have made dwelling in the past, never a healthy or desirable thing, impractical. Oh, there are scars. Depending on my mood at the moment, there are books and articles I will not read. There are scenes in television shows I will not watch, even today. The idea of miscarriage still hurts, and it always will.

Much of our healing centered around our born child. That seems to be the most frequent and most thorough remedy. But other people have seen work as a bandage for their trauma, and still others have found in this crisis an opportunity to restructure the way they live their lives, how they respond to their mates and how they look at the world—with or without future offspring. Most of the miscarriage stories I have encountered have led to strengthened faith, strengthened love, and strengthened marriages. A few have not. Any crisis exposes the weaknesses in a relationship, and when those weaknesses are significant, a crisis can tear a marriage apart. That is most unfortunate, since the pain of the miscarriage can get entangled with the pain of the divorce. Any healing after that is accomplished only with concentrated effort and exhausting self-discipline.

I think most of our healing, though, happened when we were not looking. Suddenly realizing that we had been standing near a baby in the supermarket line and had not hurt, watching a diaper commercial on television without reacting, attending someone else's baby's baptism and finding that we were not in tears—these were not goals we worked toward. They were milestones we recognized only after we had passed them.

Looking back now, I can sort out some of the understandings that accompanied these milestones. Some came sharply with clear and powerful force. Some were there, but vague, until we started trying to share them with other victims or word them for this book.

Foremost, I think, was a full and thorough realization of what really happened. There was a growing life there. Within it were all the components of a person. For some reason it stopped growing, stopped living, died. That is what really happened. It was not something different from life. It was not a *not-a-baby*. It was a tiny human being. Recognizing it as alive makes it easier to recognize it as dead.

For me this realization happened powerfully during the

course of a conference on spiritual healing. The leader launched into an exercise not unlike the one Jackie Lapa described to me. The object of the exercise was to clear the mind and allow images to form. I was tired. Tucker had been sick and wakeful and I felt like I had not slept in a week. I tried to go along with the exercise, but I seemed to be drifting closer to sleep than to involvement with the project. Then, quite unexpectedly, there was a boy-child in front of me. I had not been aware of the miscarriage in a long time. But there was my son, and he said, "I love you," with a voice I felt more than heard. At first I thought his hand was raised in greeting. Then I realized that it was nestled into a larger hand. And what shall I say about that great hand? It was that hand that, once seen, no one can say he does not recognize.

The boy-child spoke again. "May I go with Him now, please?" It was clearly something he wanted greatly. Somehow, at that moment, I knew that I had been preventing him from going.

Whether you read this story as metaphor or fact, please believe that letting go is hard. And if we are to remain healthy, it is something that we must do. But it is something that we cannot begin to do until we clearly understand what it is we are letting go of.

And it hurts. Mightily. With a pain that reaches down into the very foundation of our humanity. Trying to deny the pain is like trying to deny the dawn, or the sunset. The pain is instinctive because the loss is not a loss of something we have. It is the loss of something we are. What was it Jackie Lapa said? Cry! Scream! Whatever it takes. Get those feelings out. The fact that our child was never named, never laughed or bounced a ball or cried or said, "I love you," so that I could hear it with my ears, makes him no less a child. And me no less a parent.

Should I expect other people, people who have not been there, to understand all this? Probably not. I do know that a crisis will tell you which friends have patience and which do not.

And what of doctors? Should they be more sensitive to the emotional turmoil their activities and announcements bring on? Can they afford the emotional cost of true empathy? Should patients expect to find within the same person both the cool professional objectivity they depend on to clarify reality and the soft shoulder of a friend? Should they warn us more about the guilts and aberrant sensitivities, the suicidal thoughts, and the hormonal rebalancing? Would that just create alarm in people who may be lucky enough to have a relatively easy time? I honestly do not know the answers. I know that Jane's advice was sound: "This is a business relationship. You began it, you can terminate it." We pay too much these days to be content with less than we are paying for.

I have told many stories in these pages. There are many I left out. There was the woman who suddenly realized in the middle of her miscarriage that she was lying on the same emergency-room table where her husband had died of a heart attack two weeks before. There was the woman who was in a foreign country when she miscarried. She was required by law to name the child and buy a grave before she was allowed to go home. But there was also the woman whose miscarriage was a blessing. She had surgical scars in her uterus that would prevent her from carrying her first child. But the miscarriage cleared them away, and today she has a healthy, happy boy.

Tucker was just three days away from her second birthday when our friends Richard and Barbara miscarried. Sam and I were able to help a bit. We had been there. We had some idea of the territory, and we could tell them some of what they should expect. We were able to tell them that some of their most well-meaning friends and family would make monstrous mistakes that would hurt and anger. We were able to tell them that they were not crazy to find themselves crossing a street to avoid a playground. We were able to tell them that this pain would go on for a long time. But we were also able to tell them that most of it would go away eventually. And we were able to tell them that they would laugh again.

Out of sharing with Richard and Barbara this book was born. We were forced to clarify our understanding of what had happened to us in order to make it clear for them. In that process we found that the three most important things we could tell them were so obvious and simple that most people cannot see them. First, we could tell them that they were not alone. We had found, as they were later to find, that a surprising number of couples have experienced miscarriage. Second, we had found that most of those people do not talk about it because there is just so little to say. Finally, we were able to tell them that it does get better. Not right away and not so that you forget about it—it is never fully gone—but it does get better.

That is what this book is about. The pain of miscarriage is real and frequent and misunderstood and long and wrong and heartbreaking and no one can help it and no one can lessen it and it changes your life forever and it does get better eventually. To those who have never experienced miscarriage, this book may be useless. To those grandparents and priests and psychologists and doctors who attend the event, I hope this work will help you understand a bit more about what you are dealing with. And to those who have suffered, I hope that knowing these things, sharing them with others who have been there too, will help. That is all. If it works, that will be enough.

Related Reading

The books listed here cover all the varieties of pre- and post-natal death, including miscarriage, stillbirth, and postbirth death including crib death. Some are quite objective and technical. Some are more emotional. Most include listings of further reading, both books and articles.

Ewy, Donna, and Rodger Ewy. *Death of a Dream: Miscarriage, Stillbirth, and Newborn Loss*. New York: E. P. Dutton, 1984.

Panuthos, Claudia, and Catherine Romeo. *Ended Beginnings: Healing Childbearing Losses*. South Hadley, Mass.: Bergin & Garvey Publishers, 1984.

Peppers, Larry G., and Ronald J. Knapp. *How to Go on Living After the Death of a Baby*. Atlanta: Peachtree Publishers Limited, 1985.

Pizer, Hank, and Christine O'Brien Palinski. *Coping with a Miscarriage: Why It Happens and How to Deal with Its Impact on You and Your Family*. New York: New American Library, 1980.

Rank, Maureen. *Free to Grieve: Healing & Encouragement for Those Who Have Experienced the Physical, Mental & Emotional Trauma of Miscarriage & Stillbirth*. Minneapolis: Bethany House Publishers, 1985.

Vredevelt, Pam W. *Empty Arms: Emotional Support for Those Who Have Suffered Miscarriage or Stillbirth*. Portland: Multnomah Press, 1984.

Support Organizations

The groups listed here are peer-counseling organizations. Some have their own network of local groups and some are attached to specific hospitals. A few have hot lines for peer counseling covering the entire range of child death. Most will send reading lists and contact sheets for corresponding organizations in a specific geographic area.

AMEND
P.O. Box 2950
Hollywood, California 90028

The Compassionate Friends, Inc.
P.O. Box 3696
Oak Brook, Illinois 60522–3696

HOPE
P.O. Box 153
Florissant, Missouri 63032

HOPING
Edward W. Sparrow Hospital
1215 East Michigan Avenue
Lansing, Michigan 48909

National Sudden Infant Death Syndrome Foundation
Two Metro Plaza
Suite 205
8240 Professional Place
Landover, Maryland 20785

SHARE
St. John's Hospital
800 East Carpenter
Springfield, Illinois 62769

Support for Bereaved Parents
Houston Organization for Parent Education
14207 Locke Lane
Houston, Texas 77077

KINDER-MOURN
6900 Percade Lane
Charlotte, North Carolina 28215

INDEX

About the Author

As an actor Walter Williamson has appeared on stage in roles from Shakespeare to Neil Simon. He garnered high praise from The New York Times for his work at CSC Repertory including God in Faust and Farmer Gamon in Wild Oats. In Los Angeles where he now lives, he won a Dramalogue Award for So It Is. He has also toured his one man show, The Meditations of Four Fathers. On the large screen he is best known for several appearances with Adam Sandler including the Opera Singer in Mr. Deeds and Dandridge in The Longest Yard. As a writer Williamson has published five non-fiction books and various screenplays and plays including the upcoming True Love. He has just finished a novel set in the world of Broadway.